I STILL
Want to
Be a
Mom

I STILL Want to Be a Mom

AN INSPIRATIONAL GUIDE TO HELP WOMEN
STRUGGLING WITH INFERTILITY

SHARA HUTCHINSON

Xulon Press

Xulon Press Elite
2301 Lucien Way #415
Maitland, FL 32751
407.339.4217
www.xulonpress.com

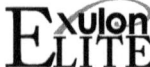

© 2018 by Shara Hutchinson

All rights reserved solely by the author. The author guarantees all contents are original and do not infringe upon the legal rights of any other person or work. No part of this book may be reproduced in any form without the permission of the author. The views expressed in this book are not necessarily those of the publisher.

Unless otherwise indicated, Scripture quotations taken from the New King James Version (NKJV). Copyright © 1979, 1980, 1982 by Thomas Nelson, Inc. Used by permission. All rights reserved.

Printed in the United States of America.

ISBN-13: 9781545641514

DEDICATION

To the child I am carrying in my womb and to any future children my husband and I will have: I love you already. You were the inspiration for this book. I never knew how strong I was until I wanted to be a mom and realized it wasn't going to be as easy to have a baby for me as it was for many other women. My desire to be a mom was greater than any pain I had to face to have you. You are valuable. You are important. You are worth it.

To all women, everywhere, struggling with infertility: Don't give up. You will be a mom!

To Jaime: I met you shortly after having a miscarriage and you shared your story with me about how you had your first son through IVF, but have been struggling to give him a sibling. You really encouraged me and gave me hope that God would bless me with a child as well, and you were right. Thank you for sharing your story with me. I pray that God grants you your heart's desire by blessing you with another child.

To George and Delcina: Trying to conceive can be an emotional rollercoaster, especially when having a baby takes much longer than expected. During this journey it is possible to experience feelings of anger, sadness, jealousy, frustration, confusion, and helplessness. Sometimes you may experience all of these in the same day. The important thing to remember is that you are not alone. You have each other. Enjoy the ride, together. Also, keep in mind there are other couples, including Todd and I, who have walked this road and succeeded. I hope our story of perseverance and achievement encourages you to maintain hope and recognize that it can happen for you too. I wish I could tell you that this road is easy, but I cannot. What I can tell you is that with God, all things are possible. Don't give up. When you think about quitting, hold on to your faith and remember why you started.

To all of the women I met on the PinkPad app: Thank you for sharing your stories with me and allowing me to follow your journeys. Even though the app is no longer active, I am glad many of us were able to keep in touch through other apps and contact methods.

ACKNOWLEDGMENTS

I went out to lunch with a friend the other day. As we sat and talked, she began to express her admiration for my determination to become a mom. She said she was impressed that I was able to experience disappointment after disappointment during this journey, yet not give up until I was a mom. She said she wished she was as strong and determined as I was. I thanked her for her compliment, but assured her that she could operate with the same tenacity by just maintaining the right mindset and surrounding herself with the right support group.

I realize that everything I have been able to accomplish during this journey is a product of not just my efforts, but those who helped encourage and inspire me along the way. I am eternally grateful for all who played a role in helping my dream of becoming a mom come to pass.

I want to thank the following individuals for their contribution to the completion of this book:

Todd Hutchinson, my husband and the father of our child and future children. One of my greatest aspirations is to serve you well as a wife, being like a fruitful vine within our house and demonstrating God's design for the role of a mother to our child(ren). Thank you for praying with me, encouraging me, crying with me, cooking for me, listening to me, and being strong for me throughout this journey. You demonstrated your commitment to the vows you made when we got married. You said "I do," and you did! During this journey, we experienced ups, downs, financial struggles, physical limitations, emotional battles, and several losses. Through it all, you never left my side, but used all of the circumstances to draw us closer together and to uncover nurturing qualities that I didn't know you had. You are everything I ever wanted in a man, and I am thankful that you are mine.

To my pastor, my father, Jeff Haygood: Thank you for modeling fatherhood so well for Todd and I. Your character, commitment, and loyalty is definitely admired. Thank you for your prayers, your listening ear, and your financial contributions. Even in times of uncertainty, you remained the voice of reason, reminding me that there is nothing too hard for God. You helped me to understand that I don't have to understand every part of God's plan. You inspired me to hold fast to my faith and not waver, knowing that He who promised is faithful. I am thankful to have you as my dad.

To my mom, Chelly Haygood: You were there throughout my entire journey to motherhood and encouraged me every step of the way. Thank you for coming to my appointments, praying with me, crying with me, and nurturing me, even at times when I thought I needed to be alone. You saw past the hard exterior and recognized when I needed to be mothered, even when I didn't recognize it. I appreciate not only your financial contributions, but genuine love for me. I am thankful to have you as my mom.

To Gina S: Whether you know it or not, you played a huge role in inspiring me to keep going in my journey after so many disappointments. Even though we only spoke online through the support groups, you offered to donate meds to me, a complete stranger, at no cost, because you knew my situation. You informed me about Starbucks benefits covering infertility and even answered all of the hundreds of questions

I had about the process. You even sent me an inspirational card, which I still have, before my third transfer for "positive vibes." That really touched me and reminded me to not lose my hope. You are such a caring person, and I am thankful to have crossed paths with you.

To Mother Winnie: Thank you for your encouragement, financial contributions, and emotional support throughout this journey. Your consistent display of love through the years really means a lot to Todd and I. We love you.

To Frank and Desirae: After our loss, you gave us a sizable, unsolicited love offering to help us purchase medications for another IVF cycle. During that time, we were wondering where the resources were going to come from. Thank you for allowing God to use you to help make our dream come true.

To Krystal Ortiz: Thank you for blessing me with a publishing package to help encourage me to birth this book. I appreciate your generosity as well as your faith that I was capable of becoming an author.

To Darryl and Mikka Abbington: You invited Todd and I into your home when you found out we were going to be doing IVF for the first time. You both shared your IVF journey and testimony about having your babies with us. You answered all of the questions we had about the process and helped us set realistic expectations. It was refreshing to hear about the experience from both the husband and wife's perspectives. I believe this equipped us for our journey. Thank you for your thoughts and prayers, as well as your transparency.

To Todd's coworkers: Several of you contributed in one way or another to make a financial contribution to help us with infertility treatments during the journey. Thank you all.

To Lashaun: Thanks for volunteering to sell candy bars to help us raise money for our first IVF cycle. I don't remember exactly how many you sold, but I know it was at least three or four shipments. I appreciate your contribution.

To Dani: Thank you for sharing your story with me, as well as giving us a rocking chair years before we were even pregnant. This was a faith-builder for me and a reminder that just because I didn't have a baby at the time, it didn't mean I wouldn't have one someday. The fact that you gave me the chair let me know that you believed that I would one day get to use it. We put the rocking chair in our nursery and during times of discouragement, I would go in the room, rock in the chair, and imagine the day when I could rock my baby in it. Thank you for your prayers and for believing that God would bless me with a child.

To my Living Word Church Family: You were with Todd and I throughout this whole journey. You prayed with us, cried with us, celebrated with us, believed with us, and contributed to us. Words cannot express what it means to serve alongside such a loving body of believers. Thank you.

To all other family and friends: Thank you for your love and support.

Finally, to my heavenly Father, Jesus Christ: the one who sees all and knows all; the one who is in control; the only wise God and savior of the world. I have truly learned that all things work together for the good for those who love you and are called according to your purpose; that there is nothing too hard for you; and that you are a promise keeper. Thank you for your faithfulness. You deserve all the glory, all the honor, and all the praise.

CONTENTS

Introduction: I am an Elephant 1

Part I: Planning

1. You WILL Be a Mom, So Plan It!. 17
2. When Things Don't Go as Planned. 36
3. Practical Principles for the Plan 49

Part II: Preparing

4. Preparing Your Body. 65
5. Preparing Your Mind. 73
6. Preparing Your Perspective. 87

Part III: Pursuing

7. Don't Forget That He WILL be A Dad 99
8. It's Time to PUSH! 106
9. Tracking Your Pursuit. 147
10. Hello Mom 239

References 245

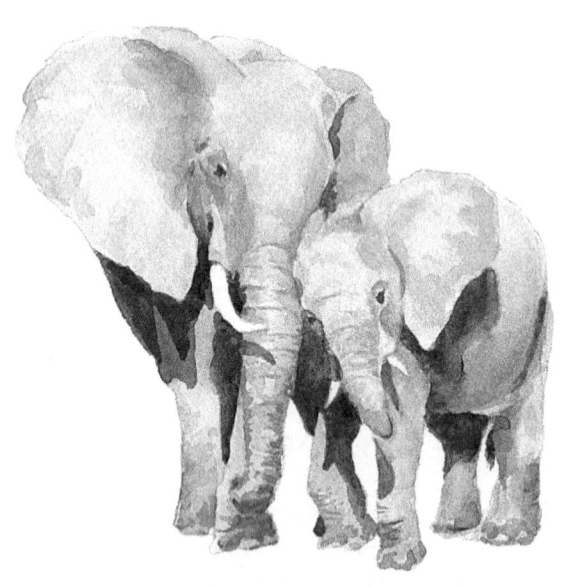

Introduction

I AM AN ELEPHANT

I never thought I'd one day be compared to an elephant; I bet you didn't think you would either. Let me explain: "An elephant and a dog became pregnant at the same time. Three months down the line, the dog gave birth to six puppies. Six months later, the dog was pregnant again, and nine months on it gave birth to another dozen puppies. The pattern continued. On the eighteenth month, the dog approached the elephant, questioning, 'Are you sure that you are pregnant? We became pregnant on the same date. I have given birth three times to a dozen puppies and they are now grown to become big dogs, yet you are still pregnant. What's going on?' The elephant replied, 'There is something I want you to understand. What I am carrying is not a puppy but an elephant. I only give birth to one in two years. When my baby hits the ground, the earth feels it. When my baby crosses the road, human beings stop and watch in admiration, what I carry draws attention. So what I'm carrying is mighty and great.'[1] In this narrative, although they started their journeys at the same time, the elephant had to watch the dog celebrate multiple births, see all of the puppies growing up, hear questions about why she still hadn't given birth yet, endure others wondering what was wrong with her, and somehow still maintain hope. Can you identify with any of that? I know I can. Throughout my journey to motherhood, I've witnessed family members, friends, coworkers, and even strangers announce pregnancies, deliver healthy babies, adopt babies, care for step-children, and ultimately be "moms," all while I sat on the sidelines waiting for my turn.

The moral of the story is the elephant had her baby when the time was right. She did not give up simply because her process took longer than someone else's. She remained confident that her baby was significant enough to wait for and used the vision of one day being a mom to inspire her to keep going, even in times where she wanted to quit. This elephant definitely represents my story; and considering you chose to read this book, I will conclude that it represents yours as well.

Who is This Book Written For?

Believe it or not, "1 in 8 couples (or 12 percent of married women) have trouble getting pregnant or sustaining a pregnancy." [4] This means that if you select eight of your female friends, family members, coworkers, or other acquaintances and line them up, at least one of them has struggled with, is struggling with, or will struggle with infertility. This book is written for women, "elephants," who fall into any of the abovementioned categories and, despite challenges, STILL wants to be a mom, whether for the first time or due to secondary infertility.

What is infertility?

According to the Office on Women's Health, "Infertility means not being able to get pregnant after one year of trying (or six months if a woman is 35 or older). Women who can get pregnant but are unable to stay pregnant may also be infertile. About 10 percent of women (6.1 million) in the United States ages 15-44 have difficulty getting pregnant or staying pregnant, according to the Centers for Disease Control and Prevention (CDC)." [2] "The inability to conceive or have a full-term pregnancy after having had children without difficulty before is the definition of secondary infertility." [3]

Why Did I Write This Book?

After compiling a list of eight surrounding couples, I discovered that my husband and I were actually the one out of eight who had trouble getting pregnant. Struggling to do something that should be so natural took us on a wild rollercoaster of emotions that has taught me some very valuable lessons that I would like to share with others. During my journey, I joined several chat groups dedicated to woman trying to conceive. I read so many stories that provided inspiration to me, and I also had a chance to dialogue with so many women dealing with this same obstacle. Even though everyone's story was quite different, one thing remained constant: we all needed encouragement. I wrote this book to inspire the women who still want to be moms to keep pursuing their dreams until they achieve them and to remind them/you that it's never too late: YOU CAN STILL BE A MOM!

— My Journey —

My husband and I met while in college. Believe it or not, we had our first date in November and were married in January. I know, I know; it was fast, but I believe when you have found the one there is no reason to delay. As of today, I have been married to my husband Todd for eight years and he is still everything I ever wanted in a man and more, so it appears my school of thought proved accurate. Prior to our union, I had a failed relationship, mainly because I chose to connect with someone who clearly did not share the same core values as I did. I settled; needless to say, it ended, leaving me time and space to evaluate my identity and draft a list of what I wanted and did not want in a husband. I outlined the negotiables and the non-negotiables. After just a couple of dates with Todd, I was able to check off the majority of my important requirements, as well as the "nice to haves". Oh and as a bonus, the items that were left, he was either working on or had the potential to accomplish, so I knew I had a winner! Everything was perfect. For the first year of marriage we were finishing up classes in preparation for graduation, so there was little to no talk about starting a family. Because my husband is a planner, he strongly encouraged me to take birth control during this time and I obliged. Finally we both graduated, found jobs in our career fields, and then bought a house. Honestly, even at that point, neither one of us was concerned about having a baby. We were enjoying having pack-up-and-send children (nieces and nephews you can pack up and send back to their parents after having fun with them). Considering all of our siblings already had children, during family events and other functions, the question always came up: "When are you two going to have a baby?" Our reply was always that we weren't sure and would begin thinking about that later on.

"Later on" didn't come until about three years into our marriage, after a routine visit to my OB-GYN. For several months I was experiencing stomach pains on my left side, which finally prompted me to discuss the issue with my OB-GYN. After some additional testing, including ultrasounds, it was determined that I had a large cyst on my left ovary that was the likely cause of this pain. My OB-GYN suggested laparoscopic surgery to remove it, since it was causing me anguish; she said it was best. I agreed, so we scheduled it for the following month. The surgery seemed to be done rather swiftly and when I woke up from the anesthesia, I was given some shocking news that was going to change my aspirations going forward. My doctor told me that once the surgical team got in there with their utensils and cameras, they discovered that I did not have a cyst. The mass that they saw on the ultrasound was actually my fallopian tubes folded and tucked behind my uterus, which meant my tubes had been unknowingly blocked for all this time. I had built-in birth control and didn't even know it.

She then gave me some great news. She said, "Although your tubes were blocked, we were able to open them and we want you to get pregnant within the next six months, just in case they re-block later." She explained that when someone has surgery to unblock tubes, the tubes are very likely to go back to their former state. I was in shock! I went from being laze-fare about having a child to instantly wanting to be a mother. If I could be completely honest, I was also relieved by the news because in the back of my mind, there was always a little uncertainty about whether or not I could conceive. There were several instances during the three years prior to my surgery that I either unintentionally or intentionally neglected to take my birth control pills and still did not get pregnant. My philosophy at the time was "If it's meant to happen, it will happen." Therefore, I was not "trying," but not consistently "preventing." Secretly, I wanted to be a mom but wasn't sure if it would ever happen, so I resolved to be content regardless. After all, I could always host sleepovers with the pack-up-and-send children. But after hearing my doctor's diagnosis, and six-month recommendation to actively try to get pregnant, a new level of excitement and hope was ignited in me. It's amazing that this one conversation, at the age of thirty, provoked a sense of urgency in me. The message, as I understood it, was ringing loud in my head: "Hurry up and get pregnant. Your biological clock is running out and you have six months to conceive." This encounter was a game-changer. My maternal instincts kicked in fast and for the first time, I could, without reservation, stand up, and declare that I WANTED TO BE A MOM!

During the next six months, I was prescribed Clomid to assist with conception because we found I wasn't ovulating on my own. The regimen was timed; it consisted of taking the pills during a certain time of my cycle and having scheduled intercourse with my husband. Sounds fun, right? Well, after six rounds of Clomid, I did accomplish something. I had six months of monitoring basal body temperature, six months of evaluating cervical mucus, six months of using ovulation predictor kits, six months of calculated sex with my husband, and then ultimately six months of negative pregnancy tests. After all this, I still wanted to be a mom.

By this point, I was confused and disappointed because I couldn't figure out why I hadn't gotten pregnant yet. After all, my fallopian tubes were open and we followed the instructions. After my six-month follow-up with the doctor, it was decided to continue this process until about a year passed with no success. I was halfway there and figured I just needed a little more time. After a year of the same outcome, I was referred to a fertility specialist. I searched my good friend Google and found Ohio Reproductive Medicine was the closest reproductive endocrinologist's office with the highest live birth rates for Columbus at the time. I browsed their website in search of the "right doctor." After reading through all of the doctors' bios that were documented and viewing their profile pictures, I felt drawn to Dr. Schmidt. Now that I had made my selection, I called and scheduled a consultation. My OB sent over all my test results, along with my past medical records and procedure details. When I walked into Dr. Schmidt's office for the first time, he made me feel hope that he would be able to, in fact, assist my husband and I with conception.

The first test he prescribed was one that I dreaded, the HSG (Hysterosalpingogram), to determine if my fallopian tubes were still open. During this procedure, he would clamp my cervix opened, shoot dye up through the vagina and cervix, and monitor the activity via ultrasound. There are only two outcomes to this test: tubes are opened or tubes are closed. This is determined by where the dye ends up. If the dye pushes through the tubes and spills over at the ends, this is considered success. If the dye does not spill over at the ends, but rather stays trapped in the tubes, this indicates failure. The procedure was pretty painful. As Dr. Schmidt vehemently attempted to push the dye through, I could tell from the image on the screen that the dye was indeed trapped. I waited for Dr. Schmidt to confirm my suspicion. He helped me up, I got dressed, and then he proceeded to share my new diagnosis. He concluded that both of my tubes were re-blocked and explained that the ONLY way that I would be able to get pregnant would be through In Vitro Fertilization (IVF). Although his bedside manner and delivery expressed compassion, in that instance my world was shattered. As soon as he uttered those words, I burst into tears. The translation I heard in my mind was "I'm sorry. You will never be able to have a baby because you don't have enough money to do IVF." Although I was discouraged, I still wanted to be a mom.

Without going into great detail on all the specifics, within a year my husband and I were able to come up with the money for the IVF process. We used savings, family and friend contributions, fundraising, and other creative methods. This was so exciting! I was going to be a mom after all. We had the initial testing done and everything looked great. My egg quality, egg reserve, uterus, ovaries, and all of the above were great. My husband's sperm count, mobility, motility, and all were great as well. Dr. Schmidt could not see any reason why our first cycle wouldn't work. We ordered all the meds; they arrived quickly, and we began the process. There were shots in the stomach (SubQ), shots in the buttocks (IM), oral medications, and a very strict calendar that had to be adhered to. I must interject that Todd was so great in all of this. He agreed to administer all of my shots, which was awesome because I knew I wouldn't be able to do it myself. So after all of the prep work, close monitoring, and the shots, we reached retrieval day. During the retrieval, the doctor uses some sort of catheter with a needle-like point, inserts it up through the vagina to the ovaries, and extracts all of the available eggs that have grown during the stimulation phase. They retrieved the eggs, mixed them with Todd's sperm, and watched them fertilize.

Next was the transfer. During the transfer, the doctor implants the fertilized embryo(s) in your uterus, on your uterine lining, with a guided ultrasound, while your bladder is full to ensure proper visibility for accuracy. When it was time to transfer, I had three great quality, five-day embryos. We transferred two into my uterus and froze the remaining one. I told everyone about our transfer and assured them all that I was indeed pregnant. I truly believed that I was, and that the IVF had worked on the first try. There was no doubt in my mind. However, on test day, to my surprise, my HCG level test returned a result of negative. When I received that phone call, my heart felt like it sunk into my stomach. My world felt like it was completely shattered once again, and

I wondered how I was going to face all of my friends and family who supported me through this journey and relay the bad news. How was I going to face my husband, who at this point was relishing at the thought of being a dad, and tell him that my body had again failed us? I mustered up the courage to tell everyone, and everyone was so understanding and encouraging. My husband was as well.

The following month, we scheduled a post-IVF meeting with the doctor to discuss what may have happened and why it didn't work on the first try, and he was just as baffled as we were. He encouraged us to try again with our last embryo for a FET (frozen embryo transfer). That is what we did. I opted to try right away, because I felt like since we could not find any contributing factors to the failed cycle, I'd just chalk it up to the fact that assisted conception is not guaranteed a hundred percent to work. I figured I had somewhere near a fifty percent chance to get my baby on the first try and since that didn't happen, the chances should be much higher with the second transfer. After having a full period, we transferred our last embryo. This time we decided not to tell anyone. We were going to surprise them with a positive pregnancy test. We transferred our remaining embryo, waited for test day, and, again, another negative test. This failure gutted me more than the first, because now we were back to square one with zero dollars in our bank account, some additional credit card debt from paying for the FET, zero frozen embryos to try again, and zero babies. Even after all of that, I still wanted to be a mom; but with no money to start over at the moment, my husband and I chose to cling closer to each other and remain thankful for what we did have.

During the next six months, we chose to enjoy life despite the disappointments. We took two vacations and then decided to assemble the baby crib that was purchased just before our first IVF cycle, in faith, to express that we still had hope. We were in this together! On August 1, 2016, my dad's birthday, I was sitting at home doing some work on the computer, and suddenly felt an inclination to go to the store and buy a pregnancy test. This feeling was unexplainable because without assisted reproductive procedures, I was aware that I was unable to get pregnant. Nevertheless, I gave in to the feeling, got up, drove to a nearby store, and purchased a First Response Early Results Test. I arrived back at home, confused about why I purchased this test in the first place, and reluctantly decided to take it. As soon as my urine touched the test applicator, instantly, I saw two lines. Up to this point I had never seen two lines, so I was in shock. I didn't know whether to scream, cry, celebrate, or assume that this test was faulty. I did all of the above and then tested again, only to discover that once again the result was positive. What a birthday surprise. I was pregnant! Despite being told that I would not be able to conceive without IVF, I was pregnant. I was pregnant naturally. At that moment, I accepted the fact that this was my miracle and I was going to be a mom after all. Within hours, everyone I could think of knew that Todd and I were having a baby, and I mean everyone. Our prayers were finally being answered. A miracle had occurred!

The next day, after the excitement wore down some and I had a chance to think soberly, I realized that I needed to call my OB-GYN and schedule my first ultrasound. It had been well over a year since I saw her, and boy was I thrilled to make my grand entrance pregnant. The appointment was scheduled about eight days later. My husband and I were over the moon excited that we were going to have an opportunity to share another "first time " together — a first positive pregnancy test and now a chance to hear our first baby's heartbeat. When the day approached, we arrived to the appointment early, holding hands and smiling from ear to ear. I enjoyed all of the nurses and staff members congratulating us, as we sat in the lobby waiting to be called. My mom was there with us, and I am not sure who was more excited: us or her. Once we got to our room, my OB greeted me with a smile and a warm welcome. She was happy that we came back pregnant. I undressed, put on the hospital gown, and then the doctor proceeded to perform the ultrasound. She moved the ultrasound speculum to the left and we didn't see anything. She explained that this was my left ovary. She then moved it over to the right slightly, and we still didn't see anything. Finally, she moved it over to the right a little more, and there was the sight we were waiting to see. There was a little baby with a strong beating heart. I could not believe my eyes. My heart had never felt such an abundance of love.

Smiles covered my mom's face, my husband's face, and mine. However, as we glanced at the doctor, her smile had turned into a look of concern. She proceeded to inform us that we had a healthy- looking baby with a strong heartbeat; however, the pregnancy was growing in the wrong place, my fallopian tubes. Our miracle had been snatched away just like that. I was experiencing an ectopic pregnancy and was scheduled for surgery the very next day. Although this was yet another traumatic experience, somehow it caused me to have more hope than I had before, because now I realized that I could actually get pregnant.

After the surgery we had very little savings, neither of my fallopian tubes (they were both removed), no baby, but a small glimmer of hope. As I sat on my living room couch the following day, that inkling of hope drove me to do the thing that always helps me overcome setbacks — devise a plan to get what I want. That's exactly what I did. I still wanted to be a mom, so I decided that I would not quit until that was my reality. As I write this introduction, I am eleven weeks pregnant, expecting to bring my baby home in October! This book is a compilation of lessons learned, inspirational thoughts, personal exercises, and planning tips taken from my journey to help you become a mom too.

How Will You Benefit From Reading This Book?

This book is broken up into three parts:

1. Planning
2. Preparing
3. Pursuing

The content is thought-provoking and very informative. I hope that after reading this book, you will be equipped with the tools necessary to formulate your personalized plan to become a mom, properly prepare your mind and body for motherhood, and exhibit the tenacity to pursue your dream until you are holding him or her in your arms.

Acronyms Used in Book

Considering each reader may be at different stages of her infertility journey and may not know some of the acronyms that will be used in this book, here is a list of some of the ones I used. Feel free to look the terms up for more information:

ANA: Anti-nuclear Antibodies
AMH: Anti-Mullerian Hormone
ART: Assisted Reproductive Technology
D&C: Dilation and curettage
FET: Frozen Embryo Transfer

FSH: Follicle-Stimulating Hormone
HSG: Hysterosalpingogram
ICSI: Intra-cytoplasmic Sperm Injection
IM: Intramuscular injections
IUI: Intra-uterine Insemination
IVF: In Vitro Fertilization
NK: Natural Killer Cells
OB-GYN: Obstetrician/Gynecologist
OHSS: Ovarian Hyper-stimulation Syndrome
OPK: Ovulation Predictor Kit
PCOS: Polycystic Ovarian Syndrome
RE: Reproductive Endocrinologist
SART: Society for Assisted Reproductive Technology
SubQ: Subcutaneous Injection
STD: Sexually Transmitted Disease
UTI: Urinary Tract Infection

My Personal Disclaimer

The content of this book is based on my personal experience, as well as the experiences of those I have had the pleasure of interacting with, throughout my journey, who were also struggling with infertility. I am not a medical professional. Use the content of this book as a guide to help you during your journey, but be sure to discuss all steps, including any vitamins/supplements you decide to take, with your doctor.

Part I
PLANNING

Chapter 1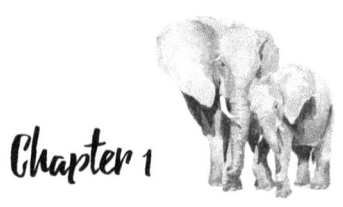

YOU WILL BE A MOM, SO PLAN IT!

As I boarded the plane, scheduled to depart at four pm, I was admittedly a little anxious because I do not fly often. I went to my assigned seat, 17B, stowed away my carry-on, and sat next to a young lady who immediately curled up in her blanket, sending me a subliminal message to keep silent during our trip. I got the hint and decided I would respect her wishes. Shortly after this encounter, the flight attendant began speaking the safety message over the intercom. She explained how to buckle the seatbelt, where to find the safety instruction pamphlet, the importance of turning off all electronic devices during take-off, and then what to do if the air pressure in the cabin gets low. She proceeded to demonstrate where to locate the oxygen masks, how to use them, and expressed that even though the apparatus will not inflate or deflate during usage, we should be assured that oxygen is flowing. One other key tip was shared during this brief, yet important, presentation: the necessity for any adult with small children to put his/her oxygen mask on first in a situation like this before assisting the child. At the time, I didn't have any children and didn't understand why someone would instruct parents to essentially help themselves first before their child. Now I understand; it is difficult and sometimes impossible to help someone with something you haven't overcome for yourself.

The plane took off in route to our destination. Midway through the flight, we began to experience a little turbulence. My blanket-covered neighbor then arose from her slumber, looked out the cabin window, and started making conversation with me. Since the ride was getting a little bumpy, I guess she felt the need to have some companionship to help ease her mind as we both traveled together. I was so glad she started talking to me, because at that moment I needed a friend to help keep me calm as well. Thankfully, we arrived to our destination safe with an on-time arrival, despite the wind and adversity.

You are now boarding a plane. As you take your seat, traveling to a destination called motherhood, I pray that through the pages of this book I can act as a friendly passenger sitting beside you, talking to you and providing you comfort to let you know that you will arrive to your destination at the appropriate time. At times, I may use these pages to teach you to "put on your oxygen mask" and learn to relax and breathe when the air seems a little thin; because after all, I had to put mine on first to be able to assist you. There will be times that the trip may get a little rocky, causing unexpected turbulence, but each word will provide some sort of reassurance that if it worked out for me, it can work out for you too!

> You will be a mom. It is not a matter of "if," but rather when and how.

You will be a mom. It is not a matter of "if," but rather when and how. Yes, let that thought sink in. You WILL be a mom. I am a firm believer that you will say what you believe; therefore, you will have what you believe. Do you believe it? Do you believe you will be a mom? If so, take a moment and boldly proclaim, "I will be a mom." If not, say it anyway because if you really want to, you will. I know you're probably wondering how I can be so confident of this without knowing your reason for infertility, or the specific details of your situation, but the truth is I don't need to have all of this information. You do.

Take a moment to reflect on your journey thus far. Think about all of your tears cried, negative pregnancy tests taken, heartaches, and all the disappointments you've experienced while trying to have a child. With all this on the forefront of your mind, write the following sentence: "I STILL WANT TO BE A MOM".

_____

_____

_____

_____

_____

Now read the above sentence out loud. Read it and re-read it until you get it in your heart.

I believe this book will be an important guide to help you win the war against infertility and position yourself to achieve your goal of becoming a mom.

Developing the Plan

I used to fantasize a lot. I'd sit back and dream about being a mom, but after trying so long the "natural way" with no success, I was unsure how I was going to get there, even though that is what I wanted. I finally realized that a dream without a plan is nothing more than a fantasy (imagining the impossible). I had to make a decision to intentionally pursue motherhood so it would actually be possible for me. You will need to do the same.

When I was in college, I was required to take several classes that at the time I thought would never be applicable to my life or career. One of those classes was called Project Management. The purpose of the class was to teach students how to create a detailed plan that would allow them to achieve a particular project, outcome, or result. I had no idea I would actually apply these very same principles to my journey to becoming a mom. The project management principles, as I remember, included documenting the following:

> I finally realized that a dream without a plan is nothing more than a fantasy

- **Desired outcome** — what you want to accomplish.
- **Milestones** — sequential list, tasks, or activities that must occur to achieve the desired outcome.
- **Risks** — things that have the potential to negatively impact or threaten the desired outcome.
- **Contingencies** — possible provisions or activities that could be implemented to address or mitigate risks.
- **Timeline** — when you would like the desired outcome.
- **Cost** — estimated budget amount needed for all milestones that make up the desired outcome.

In this next section, you will create your personalized plan. Think about this: A contractor uses a blueprint for instructions on how to build a house. The blueprint is also used to check progress and to determine when the work is completed. This plan will be considered your blueprint to baby.

Getting Started Questionnaire

We all have to start somewhere, but how do you know where to start? I'll tell you. You must evaluate where you are first. I use my phone's navigational system for directions to various places that I am unfamiliar with. The first thing I am asked, when using this program, is if the device can use my current location. If I choose not to allow the location services to track my exact coordinates, I am then asked to enter my starting address. This

> It would be impossible to provide directions to a destination without knowing the starting point.

is because it would be impossible to provide directions to a destination without knowing the starting point. This Getting Started Questionnaire is your navigation starting point. Once you fill it out and read the corresponding details, you will have enough information to document your plan using the project management principles mentioned above. The additional notes under the questions are a compilation of knowledge from my personal experiences, as well as discussions with other ladies who have struggled with infertility.

1. How old are you?
    a) 18-25
    b) 26-35
    c) 36-40
    d) Over 40

Any woman who has been trying to conceive naturally without getting pregnant after one year of trying (or six months if a woman is 35 or older) is considered infertile. This includes women who have been pregnant before, had a past live birth, or recurrent miscarriages.

2. Do you know your reason for infertility? If yes, what is it?
   a) Blocked Fallopian Tubes
   b) Diminished/low ovarian reserve
   c) Uterine Fibroids or other issues
   d) Endometriosis
   e) Male factor (low or no count, mobility, motility, shape, etc.)
   f) PCOS
   g) Thyroid problems
   h) Excess weight
   i) Ovulation or Luteal phase issues (hormone imbalance)
   j) Other health issues
   k) Unknown cause

As you can see, there are many reasons for infertility. Understanding why you are infertile is one of the first steps in addressing the root cause. If you are unsure of what has caused your infertility, there are many ways your doctor can find out. Here is a list of some:

- Performing an HSG, which uses ultrasound technology, along with a liquid dye substance, to check for blockage in your fallopian tubes. I have heard stories where women got pregnant shortly after having this test, because shooting the dye through the tubes actually cleared blockage during the procedure. This

may be the case if the blockage is minimal. If your tubes are in fact blocked, the doctor can perform laparoscopic surgery in some cases to open your tubes. This method is not guaranteed to work, but it can. If your tubes are able to get unblocked using this method, there is a chance they could re-block themselves later. If only one tube is blocked, it is possible to still get pregnant naturally, as long as you ovulate from that side.
- Drawing blood and taking urine samples to test for hormone imbalances or even some infections. If either are present, you may be prescribed medicines to address the hormone issue or infection.
- Giving either a vaginal or abdominal ultrasound to look at your ovaries and uterus. Sometimes if abnormalities are found during the ultrasound, the doctor may recommends a Sonohystogram or laparoscopy surgery to get a closer look at your reproductive system and/or remove scar tissue or other problems.
- Doing a routine pap smear to make sure there are no issues that need to be addressed. Sexually transmitted diseases and cervical issues can sometimes contribute to infertility, so it is important to get regular pap smears.
- Recommending losing weight. Being overweight can affect your fertility, so occasionally a doctor may recommend his/her patient to eat healthier and incorporate more exercise to lose some weight. I have heard stories of women who lost some weight and then got pregnant shortly after. I am not saying that losing weight will definitely help you get pregnant, but I am saying it definitely won't hurt. It's always a good idea to try to be as healthy as possible, especially for

something as physically demanding as pregnancy and delivery.
- Advising you to see a reproductive endocrinologist for further testing.
- Ordering a semen analysis for the male to check on mobility, count, and motility. Based on the results, the doctor may refer him to an urologist if necessary for further testing and treatment.
- Suggesting certain vitamins and supplements that you can take to possibly improve your reproductive functions.

3. How long have you been actively trying to conceive using no contraception?
    a) Less than 1 year
    b) 1-3 years
    c) 4-6 years
    d) 7 years or more

If you are under thirty-five and have been trying for at least a year or over thirty-five and have been trying for at least six months, it may be time to speak to your OB-GYN or a fertility specialist for possible intervention. The reason the timeframes to wait may seem so long is because every woman only has a specific window of days during a given month where she has the opportunity to get pregnant. This window occurs during ovulation. Many factors can affect ovulation. For example, if you recently stopped taking birth control after being on it for years, it may take your body a while to begin regular ovulation again, thus making it take a little longer to get pregnant. Sometimes a woman has not gotten pregnant simply because she is not having sex during her most fertile days. Regardless of your situation, you can

You Will Be A Mom, So Plan It!

seek guidance from your doctor about starting or completing your family whenever you feel it is necessary. He or she will guide you in the right direction.

4. What methods have you tried so far to get pregnant?
   a) Sex
   b) Ovulation predictor kits
   c) Basal body temperature
   d) Medications (ex. Clomid to assist with ovulation)
   e) Laparoscopic surgery (to open blocked tubes or remove cysts/fibroids)
   f) IUI
   g) IVF or other ART method

The doctors will recommend next steps on what methods to try based on your specific situation and your age. However, always do what feels right for you. Don't be afraid to get a second opinion and conduct research.

5. Have you been pregnant before? If yes, how many times and how many live births?
   a) Yes
      - Number of Pregnancies_____
      - Number of Live Births _____
   b) No

If you have been pregnant before, the good news (even if you experienced a loss) is that you know you CAN get pregnant.

6. Have you ever experienced a pregnancy loss? If yes, how many? What was the cause?
   a) Yes

I STILL Want To Be A Mom

- Number of losses_____
- Cause of loss(es) if known _____
  _____
  _____
  _____
  _____
  _____

b) No

A pregnancy loss at any stage is devastating. While you may not want to relive the thoughts of this experience, you can capture some vital information from the loss (es). If you know the cause, you can work with your doctor to see if there are preventative measures you can take in the future. If you do not know the cause, there are certain tests you may request to try and get more details to develop a plan for the next pregnancy. Here are some examples:

- Test mother for blood-clotting disorders. If you have some sort of clotting disorder, this could cause a loss after implantation has occurred. Blood thinners or other medications may be used to address this issue if found.
- Test fetal tissue from loss to see if there were any chromosomal abnormalities, which can sometimes be the cause of miscarriage. If abnormalities are found, or you have had recurrent miscarriages with no answers, you may want to request genetic testing from your doctor for you and your partner. This is a blood test that will allow you to see if your future baby is at risk of any chromosome issues. If certain genetic markers not compatible with life are found, a

genetic counselor can guide you on next steps, such as IVF with PGS testing.
- Test mother for autoimmune disorders. Certain autoimmune disorders (if left unmanaged) can cause your body to attack "foreign" cells in your body, including a fetus, causing miscarriage.
- Test mother for natural killer (NK) cells. It is believed that if these cells are present in your body, they may attack an embryo that has recently implanted, causing an early miscarriage. From what I understand, some doctors do not believe higher than normal NK cells can affect a pregnancy, but I have talked to several ladies who had multiple unexplained miscarriages who later tested positive for high NK cells, were treated, and ultimately went on to maintain a pregnancy to term. They were prescribed intralipid infusions and sometimes a certain steroid beginning in early pregnancy.
- Test to see if there is fluid buildup in your fallopian tubes. It is believed that if you have hydrosalpinx, fluid in one or both of your tubes, it can possibly leak into the uterus and negatively impact an embryo that has recently implanted. After my ectopic pregnancy, I ended up getting both tubes removed. The doctor noticed that both tubes were filled with fluid and suspected that may have been why my previous two embryo transfers failed. I have to agree because I got pregnant the very next embryo transfer once the fluid-filled tubes were gone.

6. Have you ever had an abortion?
   a) Yes
   b) No

I know this seems to be a personal question, but I believe it is one that must be addressed. Although I have never had an abortion, I know several people who have and they felt guilty afterwards. If you ever had an abortion, trying to conceive again with difficulty may cause you to get emotional and blame yourself for your infertility. Don't allow those thoughts to stay in your head. If you haven't already done so, forgive yourself and move forward. When you've had an abortion, it can affect your ability to get pregnant in the future. While it may not prevent you from getting pregnant, it may make it more difficult. Therefore, this is definitely something you want to discuss with your doctor.

7. Are you and your man both in agreement to have a child?
    a) Yes
    b) No
    c) Unsure

It is important that both you and your significant other are in agreement when trying to conceive. This process can be very emotional, and you will need each other's support during the journey. If your man is reluctant to proceed with necessary steps, try communicating with him to get to the reason why so you can address it. If you cannot come to an agreement on your own, it may be necessary to get counseling together. If one person wants to start a family and the other one doesn't, this can cause resentment in the future for either the parent who really didn't want the child and you had one anyway, or the parent who really wanted a child and was unable to try everything in his/her power to make it happen due to lack of support. After talking to several women whose men were reluctant to proceed with fertility treatments at first, here are the most common reasons why they were acting that way:

1. He was afraid he wasn't going to be a good father.
2. He felt like he wasn't ready to be a father.
3. He was afraid to get a semen analysis for fear that the issue might be him.
4. He was afraid the treatment wouldn't work and was protecting her feelings.
5. He was tired of the disappointment.
6. He was concerned about the cost.

8. Do you believe you are stable enough emotionally and financially to have a child?
   a) Yes
   b) No
   c) Unsure

Unless you are rich, I am not sure that anyone ever feels financially ready to have a child, but I know from experience that you don't have to be very wealthy to do a good job. More important than money, I believe you must be emotionally stable to care for your child. Bringing a child into chaos sometimes creates additional stress for the parents and makes the environment for the child toxic.

9. Do you have a support system or someone other than your man that you can be open with about this journey?
   a) Yes
   b) No

It was helpful for me to find a support system of women who were also going through the same thing or had already gone through the same thing with success. I downloaded several apps and joined multiple infertility and IVF chat groups where I could share my story, get feedback, and also hear the stories of others.

Feel free to follow my blog for encouraging quotes and posts. Here is the web address: istillwanttobeamom.club

10. Do you really want to have a child?
    a) Yes
    b) No
    c) Unsure

If you really want to have a child, make up your mind that no matter what obstacles or hurdles get in your way, you will give it your all. At times when you get discouraged, remember that after eight years of marriage with no baby, over six rounds of Clomid, two miscarriages, two laparoscopic surgeries, one D&C, two failed IVF cycles, one failed FET, and an ectopic pregnancy, I was able to finally get my miracle baby on my third IVF cycle! If it can happen for me, it can happen for you too. I refused to give up because even after each disappointment, I could not shake the feeling that I really wanted to be a mom. This gave me the determination to keep going!

11. What is your definition of a mom?

_____

_____

_____

_____

_____

You Will Be A Mom, So Plan It!

After being in foster homes and adopted, I realized that a mom can be more than the woman who births you. Therefore, my definition of the word mom is "a female parent who nurtures and raises a child." As I was going through my infertility journey, this was a question I had to ask myself, so I wanted you to answer it as well. Once I had *my* definition of a mom resolved in my heart, I was able to apply that to my plan to overcome infertility. I told myself that I would try everything in my power to have a biological child through birth, but if all attempts failed, I would be willing to use any method available to ensure that I had a child of my own to "nurture and raise," even if that meant using a surrogate or adoption. Your definition of the word mom will also tell you what your stopping point will be in the journey if you don't get what you want the way you want.

12. Are you willing to do whatever it takes to have a child?
    a) Yes
    b) No
    c) Unsure

If you are willing to do whatever it takes to have a child, I believe you WILL be a mom!

Your Personalized Plan to Becoming a Mom

Please answer each question:

1. What is your desired outcome?
   (Ex. To be a mom)

_____

_____

I STILL Want To Be A Mom

_____

_____

_____

2. **Based on your Getting Started Questionnaire, what milestones do you need to accomplish next to continue your journey?**
   (Ex. Request a specific test from your doctor.)

Note: As of today, what do you know needs to be accomplished in order to achieve your desired outcome? List them in order.

1) _____ Due Date _____
2) _____ Due Date _____
3) _____ Due Date _____
4) _____ Due Date _____
5) _____ Due Date _____
6) _____ Due Date _____
7) _____ Due Date _____
8) _____ Due Date _____
9) _____ Due Date _____

3. **What are the risks associated with pursuing motherhood?**
   (Ex. It might not work the first try.)

_____

_____

You Will Be A Mom, So Plan It!

_____
_____
_____
_____
_____

4. **Contingencies** — possible provisions or activities that could be implemented to address or mitigate risks. *(Ex. Begin saving extra money in case the process costs more than expected.)*

_____
_____
_____
_____
_____
_____
_____

5. **Timeline** — when you would like the desired outcome. *(Ex. Be pregnant by December 31, 2018.)*

Note: *Although you cannot put an actual "time" on when you can have your child, you can document when you would like it to happen by. You can also use this space to choose a date that you want to have all of your milestones completed.*

I STILL Want To Be A Mom

_____
_____
_____
_____
_____
_____
_____
_____
_____
_____
_____
_____

6. **Costs** — estimated budget amount needed for all milestones that make up the desired outcome. *(Ex. Estimated medication or procedure costs)*

Item	Estimated Cost	Actual Cost

Note: The plan items listed above may need to be re-evaluated and updated as you make progress towards your goal.

Journal

Write a summary of your infertility journey up to this point.

What have you learned about yourself from this journey so far?

What is your greatest strength, and how will you use that to help you achieve your goal?

Chapter 2

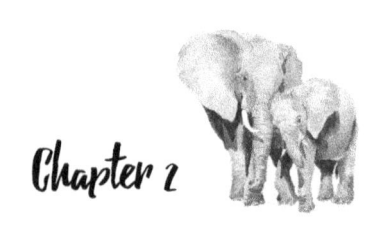

WHEN THINGS DON'T GO AS PLANNED

I opened my Gmail inbox one morning last year to two new unread emails with glaring subject lines. The first, "Welcome to Week 32 of Pregnancy," and the other "56 Days until your Due Date." I opened the first to find the following information: "This week, your baby weighs almost four pounds and could be up to 19 inches long. And though that's a head-to-toe length, your baby is actually back to a curled-up position in preparation for birth." I decided not to open the second email and simply mark it as read, because although these emails should have been helpful, they served as a reminder that I was no longer pregnant and would not be bringing my baby home next month as originally anticipated. Just a few months prior, I lost my baby boy just shy of four months pregnant. Although I had other losses and failures prior to this one, I believe this loss impacted me the most because of all the planning and preparation required to get pregnant again. I thought I had the perfect plan.

The Background Story Leading Up to the Emails

Since we had depleted our savings account and used credit cards to pay for a full IVF cycle, and then a FET cycle using the one remaining frozen embryo, we were disheartened that we still did not have a baby yet because both of those cycles failed. We were back to square one with no more embryos, no money at the time to try again, and no clue how we would afford another full round. By this point, I was aware that both of my fallopian tubes were blocked, and the only way to get pregnant would be through IVF. I was told it was impossible to get pregnant naturally, so considering we weren't in a financial position to try again, we were forced to wait. During that wait, we decided to assemble the crib that we previously purchased the year before in faith, in preparation, for our future child. This was a great bonding experience for my husband and I because as we put each piece together, we were able to talk about what it would be like when we have our future baby laying in the newly assembled crib.

About six months after we assembled the crib, I found out that I was pregnant, **naturally.** We were ecstatic! After being told that it was impossible to get pregnant naturally, we had defied the doctors and done the "impossible." Without hesitation I scheduled my first ultrasound, which based on my last period would have meant I would be eight weeks pregnant at the time of the appointment. My husband and I were overjoyed. We told everyone that we were pregnant with our miracle baby. Everyone celebrated with us, and we couldn't wait to see our little growing baby and hear that lovely, flickering heartbeat so we could bring back the good news to our friends and family. On the day of the appointment, my husband and mom accompanied me, both eager to witness the moment we had waited so long for. When it was time to go back to see the doctor, I went to my assigned room and undressed from the waist down, as instructed. The doctor came in and asked that I prop my feet up in the stirrups so she could perform the vaginal ultrasound. She inserted the instrument and began navigating around. She moved it to the left, then to the right and then to the middle. We could not see the baby.

She then looked around a little more, and then I saw the most precious sight I had ever seen. It was a little baby growing inside of me with a flickering heartbeat. As I stared at the screen, in awe, I could do nothing but smile. I looked at my husband and mom and smiled at both of them. Then I looked at the doctor's face and her smile had turned into disappointment. She proceeded to tell me that while I was seeing a perfectly growing baby with a healthy heartbeat, the baby was growing in the wrong place, my fallopian tubes. I didn't quite understand the gravity of what she was telling me, so I then asked if it was possible to move the baby from my tubes to my uterus. She explained how implantation actually works as well as why "moving" the embryo was impossible. Just then, my husband broke out into tears and my mom hugged him as he cried. I saw her wipe a few tears from her eyes as well, but at that moment I could not cry because I was in total shock. I could not believe this. How was my miracle snatched away so fast? This did not go according to plan.

I ended up having surgery the very next day to remove both of my fallopian tubes. I left the operating table unable to get pregnant naturally and this time, it really was impossible because with my tubes gone there would be no way for my husband's sperm to meet up with my eggs without intervention. The pathway was gone. I went home and had time to reflect. I decided to focus on the positive. There were three things that I was extremely grateful for:

1. I was still alive! The doctor was surprised that I was not in any pain leading up to my ultrasound, because the baby was measuring about seven weeks and had a heartbeat. She said the ectopic pregnancy could have

ruptured, causing internal bleeding, which could have been fatal. I would not have even known I was pregnant if I would not have had a "feeling" to randomly take a test, even though I didn't have any symptoms and I believed I was not able to get pregnant. This situation could have ended up a lot worse.
2. After six years of marriage, we finally had our first positive pregnancy test. Although it was ectopic, I realized that I **CAN** get pregnant. This gave me hope.
3. Even though this was a tough situation to handle, I was not alone. My husband was right there with me and we comforted each other. I realized how compassionate he was.

Instead of discouraging me, this situation encouraged me to keep going. I had a brainstorming session to figure out how we could do another cycle of IVF, and I remembered that a lady from one of my infertility support groups mentioned that she worked a part-time job at Starbucks to pay for IVF at a hundred percent. I reached out to her and she was able to answer all of my questions. Within a week of my surgery, I had figured it out. I was going to work a part-time job at Starbucks. That is how I planned to pay for it this time. I immediately filled out an application and selected the four closest Starbucks locations so I wouldn't have to drive too far if hired. The following week as I healed, I called all locations asking to speak to the store manager. It took me a while to speak with someone, but after about a week and a half of calling every day I was finally able to reach someone. Three of the stores were not hiring at the time, but the fourth was. The hiring manager scheduled an interview with me and I was so happy. I went to the interview, was hired, and then given my start date. I was officially a Starbucks partner, a barista!

Now I just had to figure out how I was going to juggle this new role with all of my other obligations:

- Being a wife to my husband (making sure I wasn't neglecting him and our house).
- I was very active in ministry at church and wanted to maintain the activities I was involved in.
- I already had a full-time job in my career field working over forty hours a week that also required me to be on-call. (My benefits package did not cover infertility treatments.)
- I was taking online classes working towards a master's degree in business administration (MBA). I was scheduled to graduate in seven months.

Needless to say, I managed to work the required average twenty hours a week at Starbucks for five months (only needed three months to be eligible), was approved for the necessary infertility coverage, started the IVF process, maintained necessary ministry functions, fulfilled my obligation at my primary place of employment, and, on top of that, graduated on time with my MBA. Everything had worked out according to plan. I do have a confession to make though. During those months, I did not give very much attention to my husband or our house. I was so tired from staying up late working and writing papers that most of our interactions included him watching me sleep. However, even though I felt bad for it, he handled it very well and was so supportive. He constantly assured me that everything was going to be alright and that he appreciated my sacrifice. He encouraged me by letting me know it would all be worth it when we were holding our baby in our arms. He also made sure dinner was made every day for us. I really learned to appreciate him even more, as he demonstrated various expressions of love for me. I know you may be wondering why he didn't work the part-time job at Starbucks. Well, he didn't because his work schedule was not as flexible as mine, so he could not guarantee that he could maintain the minimum weekly hours requirement to qualify for the benefits. I figured at least one of the readers would have that question, so I answered it for you.

I used my new benefits as soon as they were active and, just as planned, my entire IVF cycle, including meds, were paid for at a hundred percent based on the health plan I chose. The only thing I was responsible for was a few co-pays. To add icing to the cake, at the end of the treatment cycle, I took a pregnancy test and I was once again pregnant. Out of the seventeen eggs retrieved, eleven fertilized, two were transferred, and ZERO made it to freeze. The way I saw it, it didn't matter that we had none make it to freeze. Shortly after, I turned in my Starbucks apron and resigned from my position as a barista. After all, we were pregnant with another miracle baby and believed that this time we would get to bring the baby home. Everything was going perfectly. We heard the heartbeat at the first seven week ultrasound and that was such a beautiful sound, but because we had heard a heartbeat before, I contained a little excitement until our next appointment. At my thirteen-week appointment, along with hearing the heartbeat, I saw a fully formed baby. My ultrasound showed the head, body, fingers, and even toes. At that moment, I was in love. Everything was perfect, and the plan was coming together. I had no idea that within two weeks, I would have a miscarriage and lose this baby as well. I was crushed. We were crushed. All of the hard work, prayers spoken, good news shared, sleepless nights, money spent, tears cried, and moments missed with family and friends seemed to be completely in vain. My husband and I were completed devastated and were at a loss for words. How could everything look so perfect, yet provide an unexpected outcome?

Back to the Email

When I opened my Gmail inbox that morning and saw those two emails congratulating me for making it to thirty-two weeks pregnant, it was a reminder that the celebration was over and I would not have the Christmas gift hoped for on December 28th as planned, based on the original due date. Although I had other losses and failures prior to this one, I believe this loss impacted me the most because of all the planning and preparation to get pregnant again.

When Things Don't Go as Planned

Although my plan did not turn out as expected, I had to set up contingencies to address the risks and issues that had been introduced. Although this loss seemed to be unbearable at first, within two weeks of losing my baby boy I had a new plan to become a mom. No matter how bad it hurt, something in me would not allow me to give up on my dream, and I knew that the only way to look forward was to not look back.

> I knew that the only way to look forward was to not look back.

I remembered that I received a letter from COBRA to maintain the benefits from Starbucks at full-cost for a select period of time, so I searched all over the house and found the envelope. By the time I opened the letter, the deadline to pay and re-initiate these same benefits was two weeks away. The initial cost to activate them was over $1200, and the monthly payment would be about $767 to maintain. My husband and I talked and believed we could

When Things Don't Go as Planned

maintain the monthly payments if we had some help with the down payment. I don't usually ask my parents for anything, but this time we needed them. We sat down at dinner a few days later, explained the situation, along with the plan, and asked for help making the down payment. Without hesitation, the answer was yes. Even though this didn't fix the fact that we lost our baby, it was comforting to know that I have a support system to lean on beyond my husband if needed. We maintained the benefits, went through extensive testing to figure out the root cause of the loss, got cleared by the doctors to proceed, and then started IVF cycle number 3. Not only did we get to have our miracle baby this time, but we also have five frozen embryos stored away in case we want to try again for a sibling in the future. Although things didn't go as originally planned, the plan worked. None of the past pain is important to me. I am a mom.

Based on my experience, here is a list of tips on how to handle it when things don't go as planned:

1. Don't quit. I know it sounds simple, but the only way to achieve your goal is to refuse to give up until you get what you want.
2. Instead of focusing on what you can't do, try to think about what you can do. You'll be surprised by the witty ideas you come up with. This will allow you to address issues that threaten your current plan.
3. Buy something for the baby. When my husband and I purchased the baby crib, it was several years before we even had a baby to lay in it. When we assembled it a year after buying it, we still had some time before we would have a child of our own to use it. However, the act of having something in the house for our baby was a reminder that we would one day be parents. You don't

I STILL Want To Be A Mom

have to buy something as large as a crib, but even if it's a bottle or onesie, get something to help give you hope.
4. Pray and speak positively. Do not allow negative thoughts to stay in your mind or come out of your mouth. Speak what you want, not the negativity you see, and try to look at the bright side of everything.
5. Write a letter to your future unborn/unconceived child. This will allow you to express emotions that are bottled up, as well as create a happy thought of one day having a child. (**I've inserted mine at the end of this chapter**)

> Do not allow negative thoughts to stay in your mind or come out of your mouth.

6. Journal. Keep a journal of your journey so you can reflect.
7. Find other women to talk to who have been through similar situations. The success stories will remind you that it is still possible for you, and the success stories that are still in the making will remind you that you are not alone. It is important to have a support system.
8. Have fun. Do the things you love. Enjoy your friends and family. It's amazing how much laughing and smiling can heal the broken heart.
9. Read a good book.
10. Learn something new or teach yourself a new skill.
11. Clean out excess clutter from your house. When I did this, it made me feel as if I was making room for my baby.
12. Do your own research on your situation and prepare questions and/or suggestions for your doctor before appointments. Be sure to write them down in advance so you don't forget.

Journal

What was the last thing that happened to you that didn't go quite as planned? How did you handle it?

How do you handle it when things don't go according to plan? What will you do differently in the future when this happens?

What is holding you back? What will you do to prevent this from holding you back going forward?

—My Letter to Unconceived Child (7/11/2015)—

Dear…

Let's just call you baby Hutch, considering this letter was written prior to your conception.

As your dad and I prepare to begin this journey, we have so many thoughts and questions; some of which I have to mention.

Like nervousness, yet excitement…..thinking what kind of parents will we be?

Hoping we raise you to be an honorable person and wondering who you will look like, your daddy or more like me?

Will we give you all the love you need to be emotionally stable, the affection and attention?

Although I cannot answer all of my questions right now, I can tell you our sincere intentions.

First of all, we plan to give you a family foundation that neither of us experienced or had.

Being raised in the home with your biological mom and dad.

Because we have vowed to stay married forever, and we are committed to each other and God above,

And you will never have to question whether or not you were wanted because you were birthed from a calculated plan, a little science, and lots of love.

We are so excited and technically you don't even exist yet, but we have prayed and believe God, so we can rejoice.

You are definitely not an accident, but a promise fulfilled and a product of choice.

Honestly, we don't have it all figured out. Sometimes we feel like we don't have a clue.

About how to be good parents, but here is what we plan to do:

Teach you how to read and write early, and help you with your homework in hopes that you will have the highest education and knowledge.

And even though you'll likely qualify for scholarships, we'll still be sure to save money so, if necessary, we can pay for your college.

We will work hard at being good, godly examples and always make sure you go to church.

And teach you to do the right thing, simply because it's the right thing to do, even when it hurts.

We will try our best to give you all the love you need, the affection and attention

By demonstrating the love of God, whose love exemplifies perfection.

Truth is, we are still nervous and excited, and we really don't care if you look like your dad or me.

We are just happy for the opportunity to be parents and just want you to be healthy.

We promise to provide for you, protect you, and give you a childhood better than we had.

P.S. We know you'll be one hundred percent better than us.

Love,

Your Mom and Dad

Chapter 3

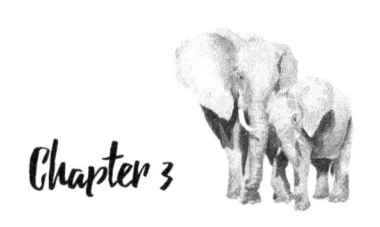

PRACTICAL PRINCIPLES FOR THE PLAN

Our principles shape our belief system. Our belief system shapes our words. Our words shape our results. Our results make up our lives. Therefore, the principles we believe ultimately affect whether or not we end up with the life we say we want. With that being said, it is important to constantly check our belief system to ensure we are well equipped to pursue our plans, even when things don't go our way. During the planning and re-planning phases of my infertility journey, I had some very exciting times and I also had some times that caused me to question my faith. During one of my down moments, I decided to encourage myself by reading stories of barren women in the Bible to see what lessons I could learn from their lives. I want to share fifteen of the practical principles with you that I believe helped shape my mindset and words to achieve motherhood. These truths not only inspired me to continue, but also gave me insight to encourage other woman who were struggling in this area as well.

1. It is important to confront your emotions and be honest with yourself. If you still want to be a mom, don't be afraid to say it.

Scripture Reference:

And He said, "I will certainly return to you according to the time of life, and behold, Sarah your wife shall have a son."(Sarah was listening in the tent door which was behind Abraham.) Now Abraham and Sarah were old, well advanced in age; and Sarah had passed the age of child-bearing. Therefore Sarah laughed within herself, saying, "After I have grown old, shall I have pleasure, my lord being old also? "And the Lord said to Abraham, **"Why did Sarah laugh, saying, 'Shall I surely bear a child, since I am old?'** Is anything too hard for the Lord? At the appointed time I will return to you, according to the time of life, and Sarah shall have a son." But Sarah denied it, saying, **"I did not laugh," for she was afraid. And He said, "No, but you did laugh!"** (Genesis 18: 10-15, NKJV)

In this scripture, I believe Sarah laughed and then denied it because she was afraid that what she heard wasn't really true, and she didn't want to get her hopes up. There have been times, especially in the beginning of my journey, where people would ask me when my husband and I were going to have a baby. Instead of telling them we were trying with no success, my response was that it really didn't matter if we had a child or not. The truth was I really did want a child, but I was afraid that it wouldn't happen; so I became comfortable with the mindset "Que sera sera (what will be will be)," instead of believing that it will be what I make it.

2. When you are struggling to conceive, it is important to pray for what you want and believe that it will happen.

Scripture Reference:
> "Now Isaac pleaded with the Lord for his wife, because she was barren; and the Lord granted his plea, and Rebekah his wife conceived" (Genesis 25: 21, NKJV).

My husband and I created a culture of prayer in our home for our future baby. This helped to strengthen our faith and strengthen our marriage.

3. Having a baby will not fix a broken marriage. It is important to get on the same page as your husband.

Scripture Reference:
> When the Lord saw that Leah was unloved, He opened her womb; but Rachel was barren. So Leah conceived and bore a son, and she called his name Reuben; for she said, "The Lord has surely looked on my affliction. Now therefore, my husband will love me" (Genesis 29:31-32, NKJV).

In this story, Leah thought that having a child would make her husband love her more. Many times as women, we feel this way as well, but that is not true. When you are going through this journey, be sure to regularly communicate with your man. Back when I was on Clomid to help me ovulate, my husband seemed to waver back and forth on whether or not he wanted a child. Since I really did, I continued to take the medication anyway, in hopes that I would get pregnant and we would live happily ever after with our child. As you know from reading about my journey in earlier chapters, the Clomid didn't work. I was actually glad it didn't because I think if I would have intentionally gotten pregnant during that time when he was saying "he wasn't ready," he may have resented me for it. Later, after more discussion, I found out the reason he was apprehensive was because he was nervous about being a dad and was unsure if he would be a good father. I assured him that he would, and through prayer and more conversations, he gained the confidence needed to be "all in" on the journey. I am so glad we were able to get that resolved before having our baby.

4. It is possible to have a baby and then struggle to get pregnant again later. Secondary infertility is real.

Scripture Reference:
"And she conceived again and bore a son, and said, 'Now I will praise the Lord.' Therefore, she called his name Judah. Then she stopped bearing" (Genesis 29:35, NKJV).

If you read the entire text, Leah stopped bearing after having four sons. I am sure this was painful to her because her body seemed to stop doing what it was once able to do. I will be honest; at first when I would read stories in my chat groups of women who had a child already, but were upset because they were struggling to have another, I would feel like they should just be grateful to already have a child. After all, there were women, such as myself, who were still waiting to have their first child and would love to be in their shoes. I realize now that assumption was wrong. All pain is real to the person who feels it, and if a woman feels her family is incomplete, she should have the right to pursue her dream

> All pain is real to the person who feels it

of having another child, no matter how many children she already has. Having a child already does not take away the hurt of disappointments and failed pregnancy tests.

5. You cannot let seeing someone else get what you want discourage you. Your time will come.

Scripture Reference:
"Now when Rachel saw that she bore Jacob no children, Rachel envied her sister, and said to Jacob, 'Give me children, or else I die!'" (Genesis 30:1, NKJV).

It is inevitable. A family member, friend, co-worker, associate, or someone around you will get pregnant while you are still trying. You cannot get so focused on this that you lose sight of your journey. If you believe it will happen for you, you will still be able to rejoice with them. If you don't believe it will really happen for you, their pregnancy can serve as a dagger in the heart that plagues your mind with thoughts that tell you you'll never have a child but everyone else will. Choose to believe that it will happen for you when the time is right, if you do not quit, and I assure you, it will. When I got pregnant with my ectopic, my sister-in-law had recently found out she was pregnant as well. She went for her ultrasound and everything was fine. When I went for my ultrasound about a week or so after hers, I found out that my baby was growing in my tubes and I needed to have surgery to terminate the pregnancy. Even though it wasn't my turn yet, it didn't make her pregnancy any less special. I was still happy for her.

6. Sometimes you may have to be willing to use unconventional methods to get what you want.

Scripture Reference:
> So she said, "Here is my maid Bilhah; go in to her, and she will bear a child on my knees, that I also may have children by her." Then she gave him Bilhah her maid as wife, and Jacob went in to her. And Bilhah conceived and bore Jacob a son. Then Rachel said, "God has judged my case; and He has also heard my voice and given me a son." Therefore she called his name Dan. And Rachel's maid Bilhah conceived again and bore Jacob a second son (Genesis 30:3-7, NKJV).

Since Rachel could not conceive, she was willing to use a "surrogate" to have a baby. She wanted a child so bad, she didn't care what she had to do to have one. I have talked to several women who needed to use a surrogate, use donor eggs, sperm or embryos, or even adopt to become a mom. When you are going through this journey, it is important to determine how far you are willing to go to have a child. You have to ask yourself: does carrying the child or the child carrying your DNA make you a mom, or is a mom more than that? There were a couple times after heartaches that we considered other options. If I would have made it to the end of my rope without having a child, I was willing to either adopt, use a surrogate, or use whatever other method that would have given me a better chance of being a mom. While these were held in the

Practical Principles for the Plan

back of my mind as absolute last resorts, I did have discussions about them with my husband and family in the event my journey would take us that far.

7. Use your past success of conceiving and birthing a child to predict future success. There is hope to have a baby after secondary infertility.

Scripture Reference:
"And God listened to Leah, and she conceived and bore Jacob a fifth son" (Genesis 30: 17, NKJV).

In the fourth point above, Leah had stopped conceiving after four sons. She prayed and eventually she was able to conceive again. Remember, if you had a child before, it is possible to have another one, even if it takes you longer to get pregnant. I have talked to ladies who have had a tubal ligation reversal, or their husbands got a vasectomy reversal after remarrying. In some cases, the process worked and they got pregnant naturally. In other cases, they needed to use an ART method to get pregnant.

8. Know that no matter how long you wait, it is still possible to have your child if you don't quit.

Scripture reference:
Then God remembered Rachel, and God listened to her and opened her womb. And she conceived and bore a son, and said, "God has taken away my reproach." So she called his name Joseph, and said, "The Lord shall add to me another son" (Genesis 30:22-24, NKJV).

9. In preparation for pregnancy, be careful what you put in your body. Be sure to get the right vitamins and nutrients.

Scripture Reference:
> And the Angel of the Lord appeared to the woman and said to her, "Indeed now, you are barren and have borne no children, but you shall conceive and bear a son. Now therefore, please be careful not to drink wine or similar drink, and not to eat anything unclean. For behold, you shall conceive and bear a son. And no razor shall come upon his head, for the child shall be a Nazirite to God from the womb; and he shall begin to deliver Israel out of the hand of the Philistines" (Judges 13:3-5, NKJV).

I have been a part of many discussions where women wonder if it is necessary to stop drinking alcohol, smoking cigarettes, or eating unhealthy foods in order to get pregnant. I don't know if cutting those things out will help you get pregnant, but I do think that it wouldn't hurt your chances. I believe it is better to rid your body of toxins that could potentially harm you or your future child while trying to conceive. In fact, if you research, there have been many studies done to show that these items can affect the reproductive system.

10. Pray and think about what you will do as parents.

Scripture Reference:
> "Then Manoah prayed to the Lord, and said, 'O my Lord, please let the Man of God whom

You sent come to us again and teach us what
we shall do for the child who will be born'"
(Judges 13:8, NKJV).

It's never too early to learn about being a parent. I read articles, listened to inspirational videos, and talked to other parents while preparing to be a mother. While you can never truly be prepared to be a parent, or know everything about raising a child, you can learn some valuable lessons that will help you some day.

11. Try to imagine what it will be like when your baby is born instead of focusing on fear.

Scripture reference:
But the angel said to him, "Do not be afraid, Zacharias, for your prayer is heard; and your wife Elizabeth will bear you a son, and you shall call his name John. And you will have joy and gladness, and many will rejoice at his birth" (Luke 1:13-14).

Positive thoughts create a positive attitude. Don't allow fear to stop you in pursuit. Trust that you will be a mom and allow that thought to give you lasting joy.

12. If you aren't going to speak positive, don't say anything. Do not allow people to speak fear or doubt into your mind.

Scripture Reference:
"But behold, you will be mute and not able to speak until the day these things take place,

I STILL Want To Be A Mom

because you did not believe my words which will be fulfilled in their own time." And the people waited for Zacharias, and marveled that he lingered so long in the temple. But when he came out, he could not speak to them; and they perceived that he had seen a vision in the temple, for he beckoned to them and remained speechless (Luke 1:13-14, NKJV).

Infertility is a tough journey. Sometimes people won't know the right words to say, and neither will you. Try to refrain from speaking doubt and disbelief because this will affect your attitude and motivation. Try to find a positive in every negative situation.

13. It's not a matter of if it will happen or how it will happen; just know that it will happen.

Scripture Reference:

Then the angel said to her, "Do not be afraid, Mary, for you have found favor with God. And behold, you will conceive in your womb and bring forth a Son, and shall call His name Jesus. He will be great, and will be called the Son of the Highest; and the Lord God will give Him the throne of His father David. And He will reign over the house of Jacob forever, and of His kingdom there will be no end. Then Mary said to the angel, "How can this be, since I do not know a man?" (Luke 1:30-34, NKJV).

> Try to find a positive in every negative situation.

Don't be so concerned about the when and the how; just focus on the fact that it will happen. This principle helped me stay encouraged throughout my journey.

14. Don't give up just because of your age. Know that if it can happen for someone else, it can happen for you too.

Scripture Reference:
"Now indeed, Elizabeth your relative has also conceived a son in her old age; and this is now the sixth month for her who was called barren. For with God nothing will be impossible" (Luke 1:36-37, NKJV).

It's never too late, so don't give up. I thought that I needed to have a baby before I was thirty, but that didn't happen and I am just as happy. I actually got better embryos my last IVF cycle than I did on my first. Also, while there are advantages to having a child when you are younger, honestly I am glad to have a child a little later because we are much more stable now than when we were in our twenties. You don't need to have a child by a certain age, just because society tells you to.

> Don't be so concerned about the when and the how; just focus on the fact that it will happen.

15. It is important to have a strong support group and socialize with others going through the same thing and have already been through it.

Scripture Reference:
> And it happened, when Elizabeth heard the greeting of Mary, that the babe leaped in her womb; and Elizabeth was filled with the Holy Spirit. Then she spoke out with a loud voice and said, "Blessed are you among women, and blessed is the fruit of your womb! But why is this granted to me, that the mother of my Lord should come to me? For indeed, as soon as the voice of your greeting sounded in my ears, the babe leaped in my womb for joy. Blessed is she who believed, for there will be a fulfillment of those things which were told her from the Lord." (Luke 1: 41-45, NKJV).

When you communicate with ladies that have had similar struggles and have overcome, it encourages you. I joined several infertility/IVF apps and support groups to have this type of interaction. When no one else understood what I was going through, they did. Having that support system was key to keeping me on the path. I watched so many ladies have several failed attempts and then finally get their "rainbow baby." I used their stories as inspiration until mine became one of the success stories on the wall as well.

Practical Principles for the Plan

◈ Journal ◈

What inspires you to keep going when you feel like quitting?

What is your biggest fear? What thoughts will you use to overcome it?

Write out three things you are most thankful for and why.

Part II
PREPARING

Chapter 4

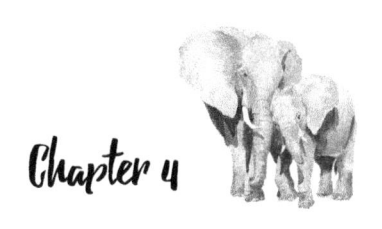

PREPARING YOUR BODY

I have a confession to make: I absolutely love food. I can eat all day every day. One of my favorite channels on YouTube is a cooking show called "Tasty." Sometimes my husband and I watch that channel for hours to get ideas on new meals to make. Well, let me clarify — to get ideas on new meals for him to make. Although I enjoy pleasuring my palette with a variety of meals and desserts, I do not like to actually prepare the meals. My husband took over the role of the house chef a few years ago because he said he wanted "good food." Apparently, the food I was throwing together over the past five years was not good enough for him. He wanted freshly chopped vegetables, carefully seasoned poultry, beautifully garnished dishes, and homemade desserts. I wanted that too; I just wanted to be able to snap my fingers and make that happen. Unfortunately, I discovered my idea was not realistic, so needless to say, he took over the kitchen and now we have a win-win situation. We both get to eat "good food," and I don't have to make it.

When I first figured out that I was ready to get pregnant, I took the same approach with my body as I did with my cooking. I felt as if I could just snap my fingers and have a baby; however, it wasn't quite like that. The very first test

I had done starting out was the 21-day progesterone test to determine if I was ovulating; I was not. If your progesterone is too low at that point, it suggests that you didn't ovulate and mine was, so it indicated that I didn't. I wanted an easy fix, but how was I going to get my body to cooperate and do what it was designed to do, make a baby? After speaking to my doctor, I was advised that while I could be given a medication called Clomid to help me ovulate, it would be advantageous to prepare my body for conception and pregnancy considering many factors play a role in fertility. He gave me several tips, but to be honest, they all sounded similar to carefully chopping up peppers and onions and making a fancy dish. He even suggested I should exercise and get to a healthier weight. Why couldn't I just go to the grocery store and purchase a fully-cooked frozen meal with freshly chopped peppers and onions already in it, and then act as if I made it from scratch? Why couldn't I just eat one salad and lose all the weight the very next day? Why couldn't I just pop a pill and then pop out a baby? I guess because life doesn't work that way. Just as you can taste the difference between a homemade meal and a store-bought, frozen meal, my doctor could tell that I had not put any effort into getting my body ready to get pregnant. He did not tell me that I would not get pregnant if I did nothing, but he just said my chances would increase if I did. I knew he was right and even though it would take time, I decided to put in work to increase the possibility of getting pregnant.

Since you are in the process of trying to have a baby, I would like to share information with you about preparing your body. I want you to really think about whether or not you are giving your body the best possible chance of conception. Whether you are trying naturally, taking medicine to help with ovulation, doing an IUI, IVF, or FET, all of these tips will be good for you to implement while you are on your journey, but ideally you should start thirty to ninety days prior to trying to conceive.

Overall Health

- Start taking a daily prenatal vitamin. If it has folic acid (folate) in it, that is a plus. If not, take folic acid separately.
- Eat healthy meals daily. This includes a well-balanced diet with fruits vegetables, whole grains, and proteins. Try to eat every few hours and, if possible, don't skip meals.
- Exercise. You don't have to do vigorous activities. Even taking short walks daily will help increase your blood flow.
- Quit smoking, drinking alcohol, and using any non-prescribed drugs.
- Drink plenty of water each day. I believe my doctor said to drink at least eight cups of water a day.
- Limit caffeine intake.
- Be sure to keep in contact with your doctor on any changes you are making or supplements you decide to take.

Egg Quality/Uterine Lining Support

During my first two egg retrievals for IVF, I did not get very many good quality embryos. After some research and chatting with other ladies from infertility groups, I learned about a few ways to help ensure my egg quality and uterine lining were better. I believe applying that knowledge helped me get a better result the last time. On my third IVF, I was three years older than when I had my first IVF, and I got more good quality embryos and even had a great amount make it to freeze. While I did opt to do ICSI that time, the other changes I made, in addition to the above, was taking the following a few months before starting the cycle:

- Ubiquinol/CoQ10
- DHEA
- POM (Pomegranate) juice
- MACA root
- Royal Jelly

Note: These are just supplements I took. You may need a different combination or some that are not on my list based on your body. If you have already been diagnosed with a diminished egg reserve or egg quality, I recommend reading a book called "It Starts with the Egg" by Rebecca Fett to assist with improving egg quality. Several ladies from my infertility support groups had this issue, followed the instructions in this book, and got results. I did not actually read the book because my AMH and FSH levels were within normal range when tested, indicating my egg quality and egg reserve were good and not diminished; but I wanted to suggest it for anyone reading this book who has a known issue in this area.

Next Steps

What do you need to do to prepare your body for conception?

_____

_____

_____

_____

Preparing Your Body

What are you going to do to better prepare your body for conception?

Do you have an accountability partner to make sure you stay on track? If so, who is it? If not, find one. It is important that you share your goals with someone who will make sure you are on track, even when you feel like quitting.

_____

_____

_____

_____

_____

_____

_____

_____

_____

Write down three goals. Put reminders on your calendar for the due date(s) to make sure you achieve them.

    1. I will _____

_____

_____

_____ by this date

_____ .

Preparing Your Body

2. I will _____
   _____
   _____
   _____
   _____ by this date
   _____ .

3. I will _____
   _____
   _____
   _____ by this date
   _____ .

Journal

What do you like best about yourself?

Do you usually achieve your goals? If not, why?

What keeps you pursuing motherhood even when you feel like quitting?

Chapter 5

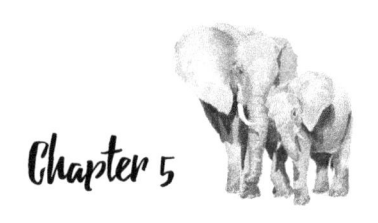

PREPARING YOUR MIND

It was 4:55pm on a Friday. I received an unexpected meeting invite from my manager for a meeting scheduled to take place in twenty minutes. The description was blank, but that subject just read "Quick Discussion." I thought what do we need to have a quick discussion about? What was so urgent that it could not wait until Monday? My mind started wandering, wondering why I would receive a random invite at the end of the business day, on a Friday, for that same day. The first thought that came to my mind was that I was getting fired, but I didn't know why. I instantly started trying to figure out what I was being terminated for. I could not recall anything specific that happened recently to cause this, so I was confused. I was terrified, so in preparation to go to my managers' office, I did what anyone in my predicament would do— I started packing all of my belongings from my office in boxes so when they walked me out it would be easier. I even took down the pictures I had tacked to my wall. I finished getting my stuff packed about 5:10, and I then sent my team an instant message letting them know I appreciated all their hard work and was grateful to work closely with such great people. After all, I didn't want to leave without giving a few last words of recognition for their efforts.

Once the clock struck 5:13, I left all of my boxes on the top of my desk and headed to my manager's office. I walked in the doorway and my eyes opened as wide as saucers, because our CEO was also sitting there. I felt the biggest lump in my throat as I took a large gulp. My heart sunk in my chest and I felt even more nervous, so I quickly took a seat. They both looked at me and the conversation began. They called the meeting to inform me of some positive organization changes that were going to be taking place in the near future for my department, to better prepare us to handle the company's continued growth and wanted me to know in advance. They also wanted to get my input about some of the proposed changes. My eyes went back to their normal size, I gladly picked my heart up from the floor, the lump in my throat dissolved, and then I was able to respond with my input. The meeting went well.

As I walked back to my office, I was hoping no one had stopped by while I was out and seen the boxes. I felt so stupid. I had assumed that an unexpected meeting held at the end of the day meant termination was eminent. I was completely wrong, and now I couldn't just leave the office by 5:30 as planned. I had to stay over, unpack all my stuff, and redecorate as if nothing ever happened.

How did one meeting request translate a message to me that I was getting fired? I know you're probably wondering the same thing. Well, it's pretty simple. My mind started going down a negative path, and I allowed it to spiral out of control to create a scenario that wasn't even real. This caused me to take action that was unnecessary out of worry and fear. This goes to show you that our thoughts are powerful. One negative thought can disrupt your whole mood and cause you to be fearful, depressed, or anxious, if you let it. On the other hand, one positive thought spoken over and over will create a positive mood and outlook, causing you to have the tenacity to keep chasing after your dream until you achieve it.

When dealing with infertility it is very easy to expect the worst, especially when you have experienced disappointment after disappointment. Then when it is time to take steps towards your goal, you may create a scenario in your mind that disrupts your mood and your pursuit. It can cause you to be more sensitive to comments made or other emotional triggers. Therefore, if you want to be a mom, it is important to prepare your mind for the inevitable fight against pessimism. You cannot necessarily stop the negative thoughts, but you can persistently combat negative thoughts with positive ones.

Prepare Your Mind

When I was in high school, I was on the track-and-field team. I ran only short distances or sprints. I participated in the 200-yard dash as well as the 4x200 relay. I did not have the endurance or the motivation to run long distance. Running long distance, more than one mile at a time, required a different level of training. Sprints were over very quickly, so the main thing you had to do to finish was to maintain a fast speed thorough the race, and then save some energy to pick up the pace a little toward the finish line. The long-distance runs, however, required keeping a steady pace throughout the race and then preparing yourself to sprint at the end. If you sprinted in the beginning, there was a good chance you would run out of energy before the end. That is why it was important to find the appropriate pace for yourself.

> You cannot necessarily stop the negative thoughts, but you can persistently combat negative thoughts with positive ones.

During a long-distance run, you are more likely to quit because you have what seems to be a far way to go. The only way to ensure you get to the finish line is to train your mind to push yourself, even when your body wants to give up. This journey with infertility is definitely more of a long-distance run, even a marathon, than a sprint. There will be times when your goal of being a mom, the finish line, seems so far away but you want it to happen quickly. You may see other "runners" or women in the same race have their babies before you, but you cannot get distracted by that. It is important to maintain a healthy pace for yourself, because you don't want to run out of energy before reaching the goal. No matter what happens along the way, if you have predetermined in your mind that you will not quit, you won't, even when you experience fatigue and other physical ailments. If you are going to be a mom, you must learn to control your thoughts.

One of my favorite quotes is this: "The greatest weapon against stress is our ability to choose one thought over another" – William James.[6] I really believe this to be true and it really helped me. When I used to have thoughts of doubt, I read through all the success stories of women who had multiple failures, and then finally got their babies and didn't quit. Then I thought to myself, if it can happen for them it is still possible for me. One of my greatest motivations to continue my pursuit of being a mom was seeing the results of others, and praying and knowing that my time was coming!

Here are tactics you can use to train your mind to choose positive thoughts over negative thoughts:

- Pay close attention to what you are thinking about. When a negative thought arises, find a positive one to counteract it. For example, when I was going through my second IVF cycle, I had moments where I reflected

Preparing Your Mind

on the fact that my first one failed and I thought to myself, "What if this one fails too?" Instead of dwelling on that negative thought, I decided to focus on the "now" and think about the fact that I had a chance to try again. I then asked myself a new question: "What if it actually works this time?"
- Find something to be thankful for every day. It's hard to keep a positive mindset when you only focus on what's going wrong.
- Try to look for the positive in every situation. After having my ectopic and getting both fallopian tubes removed, I was a little upset that I would never be able to get pregnant naturally. Instead of focusing on that, I realized that the bright side was that I still had my uterus and ovaries, so I could still get pregnant; I would just need intervention each time. Then I thought of another positive: after having my babies, I would not have to worry about what type of birth control I was going to use because after all, I wouldn't need it.

> Learn to control your emotions.

- Learn to control your emotions. Never make an important decision while you are very emotional (too sad, too happy, and too angry). Decisions made during these times are usually regretted because we didn't think all the way through them.
- Focus on the facts and ignore the lies.
- Speak positively about your situation. Read the **Future Mom Mantra** (located at the end of this chapter) out loud every morning when you wake up and at night before you go to bed. If it helps, read it while looking in the mirror. You are more likely to remember and believe what you speak out loud.

- Surround yourself around people who inspire you.
- Listen to motivational talks.
- Read motivational stories and books.
- Encourage someone else who is going through a tough time.

Important Note: If you are constantly dealing with thoughts that you cannot control, and find yourself to be sad or depressed all of the time, I would recommend seeing a counselor or talking to your doctor about your feelings. Sometimes you may need additional assistance getting through these challenges.

Handling Emotional Triggers

In this next section, I have listed some emotional triggers and responses, as well as a combatting thought that you can choose instead of the negative one.

1. **Thought**: My coworker, family member, or friend announces her new pregnancy and I still haven't had a child yet.

Response: Learn to celebrate with others. Just because you haven't had your child yet, it doesn't mean it won't happen for you. If you are getting overwhelmed with pregnancy posts on social media, you may want to stay off of social media for a while until you think you are emotionally ready to handle seeing them.

2. **Thought:** I feel like my friend or family member is in competition with me. I announced that I am struggling

Preparing Your Mind

to get pregnant, and now my friend or family member announces that she is pregnant.

Response: It could be a coincidence. While there are some people that may have malicious intent, don't let that be the first conclusion you jump to. Remember, sometimes our emotions can cause us to read more into situations because of the way we feel about our situation. On the other hand, even if they are "showing off" that they can get pregnant, it won't change anything for you. You just have to remember that your time is coming, and your baby will be so loved because of all you had to go through.

3. **Thought:** Someone who has not struggled as long I have is complaining about trying to conceive.

Response: All pain is real to the person who feels it. Just because they haven't waited as long as you have, it doesn't mean that they are not frustrated in their own way.

4. **Thought:** I had a miscarriage, but I should be due next month or this day would have been my baby's birthday.

Response: Whenever an important day like one of these examples arises, no one can tell you how to feel. If you want to celebrate the day, celebrate the life you had growing inside of you. If you choose to not acknowledge the day, that is also completely up to you. If you know you get emotional around that time, it may be good to schedule a vacation or outing with friends and family during that date so you can have fun and enjoy the moment.

5. **Thought**: You see someone holding her baby and you want one.

Response: Instead of allowing feelings of jealousy or despair to arise in you, try to use that as an opportunity to imagine what it will be like for you when you are holding your baby someday.

6. **Thought:** It seems to be so much easier for others to get pregnant (someone you know gets pregnant the first month of trying).

Response: While this may be true, don't allow it to discourage you. You will have your baby in due time.

7. **Thought**: You were pregnant with someone, and you lost your baby and she didn't.

Response: Although it may be hard for you to celebrate with her after your loss, you have to remember that the life this person is carrying is precious as well. Take your time to grieve, but try not to make the other person feel guilty that she didn't lose her baby as well. This may be an emotional situation for both woman involved. I'm sure the other lady feels bad and does not know how to interact with you and celebrate around you, while still considering your feelings and emotions.

8. **Thought:** You see someone who takes her kids for granted, or mistreats them, get pregnant again.

Response: You cannot control what anyone else does, but you can control the type of parent you will be.

9. Thought: Someone complains to you that she is pregnant.

Response: Most of the time if a woman is upset about being pregnant, it is because her situation is not conducive to having a child, it was an "accident," or there are issues going on with her and the child's father. When going through fertility treatments, your baby is never an accident because the pregnancy is planned, and you and your man both want the child and are working together to make it happen. Therefore, don't even compare your situation to hers. Try to be compassionate because there is heartache in both of your situations, just for different reasons.

10. Thought: Someone you know gets an abortion while all you want is to have a child.

Response: You cannot control what anyone else does, but you can decide that is something that you would not do.

—Future Mom Mantra—

Today, I am happy because I am one step closer to being a mom than I was yesterday.

I realize that this journey is a marathon, and not a sprint, so I will exercise endurance until I am holding my dream.

Despite what I have been through up to this point, I still want to be a mom.

I am willing to fight for my dream, overcome obstacles for my dream, and push past fears for my dream, so I can live my dream…my dream of becoming a mom.

No matter what steps I have to take to get there, I am willing because when this journey has ended, and I am holding my baby in my arms, I know that it will all be worth it.

Therefore, I am going to be happy throughout this journey.

I am going to be thankful throughout my journey.

I am going to be positive throughout this journey.

I am going to take care of my body, eat right, and get proper rest throughout this journey.

I am actually excited about this journey because I know it's not a matter of "if it will happen," but rather a matter of "when it will happen."

I know it's not a matter of if it will happen, but rather a matter of how it will happen.

Since I know that it will happen, I can trust the process and keep moving forward, even when things don't always turn out how I want or expect them to.

I still want to be a mom.

I know I am going to be a good mom.

I am fearfully and wonderfully made.

Preparing Your Mind

I am already equipped with all of the skills and abilities to do anything I put my mind to.

I am going to enjoy every moment of this journey and one day, when my baby is old enough, I will tell him or her about how much I wanted to bring him/her in this world.

I have fought so hard to get to this place and I will not let anything discourage me.

I will not complain.

I will not focus on past failures.

I will not speak negatively because I realize that my words shape my mood.

I will not worry because I realize that my worries are usually about situations that are beyond my control.

I will not be afraid because I realize that my fears are usually about situations occurring that haven't even happened or won't happen.

I know that fears are fake exaggerations affecting my reality and I will not allow myself to concentrate on them.

I will practice replacing negative thoughts with positive ones until it gets easier and easier to think positively.

I will not be down.

I will not be depressed.

I will not blame myself.

I will not blame my body.

I will not blame others.

I will choose joy instead of pain.

I will choose love instead of fear.

I will choose expectation instead of worry.

I will do what I can and not worry about what I can't.

I will surround myself with people who encourage me and promote positivity in my life. When no one else is around to encourage me, I will encourage myself.

After all, I have been able to make it this far.

Nothing can stop me. I am a conqueror.

I am strong. I can do this.

I will survive this journey.

I will have a healthy pregnancy.

I will deliver a healthy baby.

I will have a happy, healthy, and safe delivery.

I will get to take my baby home with me this time.

I can't wait to hold my baby in my arms for the first time.

This thought makes me smile because as I say this, I am literally visualizing my baby in my arms. Wow, MY baby in MY arms.

My heart is smiling. My face is smiling. The hope I feel overpowers any negative thoughts.

Today, I am happy because I am one step closer to being a mom than I was yesterday.

I realize that this journey is a marathon, and not a sprint, so I will exercise endurance until I am holding my dream.

Despite what I have been through up to this point, I still want to be a mom.

I am willing to fight for my dream, overcome obstacles for my dream, and push past fears for my dream so I can live my dream... my dream of becoming a mom.

I still want to be a mom.

Journal

Why do you get upset when friends, family, and coworkers announce their new pregnancies?

Are you embarrassed about your struggle with infertility? If so, why?

Do you believe you will get to be a mom someday?

Are you ready to start or continue this journey?

How can you remain positive when you get negative results?

What thought(s) causes you to get discouraged? What will you do to combat those thoughts?

Chapter 6

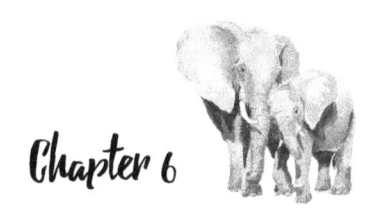

PREPARING YOUR PERSPECTIVE

It's amazing how two people can stare at the same glass that has water in it. One will see the glass full, while the other sees the glass as half empty. One has sight, while the other has vision, but which one is most important to have? I believe Helen Keller, a woman who was left blind and deaf after a childhood illness in the 1800s, answered this question. She said, "The only thing worse than being blind is having sight but no vision."[5] Despite her disabilities, she was known for being "one of the most prolific authors, political activists and lecturers"[5] of her time. I learned about Helen Keller when I was in elementary school and admired her tenacity. I wondered how she accomplished all of her achievements and made history considering her circumstance. It wasn't until I was grown that I understood how vision really worked. Helen always saw the "glass half full" because she had the proper perspective on life. Although people saw her situation as being unfortunate, she saw her situation as being an opportunity; an opportunity to make a difference, despite her natural

> If you focus on the positives in life, the negatives will not be able to stop you from accomplishing whatever you want to accomplish.

limitations. She saw her disabilities as opportunities to show others that if you focus on the positives in life, the negatives will not be able to stop you from accomplishing whatever you want to accomplish. She recognized that being physically blind was not as bad as not being able to dream, imagine the future, or plan for a better tomorrow.

Helen knew that having vision was much more valuable than having sight, because sometimes our sight can skew our vision. This happens when we look at a situation or problem with our natural eyes, but cannot see beyond it to find a solution, meaning our perspective is off.

When battling infertility and pursuing motherhood, it is important to make sure you have the right perspective, because perspective determines attitude and attitude determine actions. When your perspective is not right, you become so paralyzed by the "what ifs" that you will be reluctant to keep moving forward, when faced with the various obstacles this journey may uncover. If you are going to achieve the desired outcome, you will need to be able to look past the negative and see the positives; so you can use your vision of one day becoming a mom to give you the drive and determination to keep going, even when you feel like quitting.

Principles for the Proper Perspective

1. Always look at the bright side.
2. Don't blame yourself for your infertility.
3. Know that happiness is not a product of what happens, but rather a choice.
4. You must celebrate each victory, no matter how small.

5. Everything is not drama-worthy, so choose your battles.
6. Focus on what you want, not what you see.

While I used the above principles to help shape my perspective during my journey, I also used the success stories of others to give me a vision of what was possible for me if I decided not to quit. When I would experience failures or feel discouraged, I would think about women I had encountered in my life from support groups or through friends who had challenges getting pregnant or having a baby, but eventually became moms. Their outcomes gave me hope.

I have included some of the stories that I held onto until it was my turn to become a mom. Feel free to read them and begin seeing your glass as half full. Know that if it happened for them and for me, it can happen for you too!

Each story expresses a type of perspectives needed for success:

1. There is no limit to how far I will go to become a mom.
2. I will do whatever it takes to become a mom.
3. I will not allow negative news to cause me to abort my dream of becoming a mom.
4. It only takes one good embryo to have a healthy baby.

—Success Stories—

Story # 1: There is no limit to how far I will go to become a mom.

Gina S. and her husband had their first appointment with an RE in 2011. After some testing, she found out that she had endometriosis, high FSH (14), and MTHFR Mutation. She told me that MTHFR is a genetic issue that can cause infertility, recurrent miscarriages, or other birth issues. In 2012, she had laparoscopic surgery to treat the endometriosis. She then did six IUIs and, unfortunately, all six failed. Now it was time to move to IVF. After checking prices in the states, they decided to do IVF abroad in Prague at the clinic called Gennet; IVF there cost $7,000. They stayed in Prague for two weeks and used that time to not only pursue their dream of being parents, but to also catch up on some much needed rest and relaxation.

In July 2013, she was pregnant from this cycle and went on to have a beautiful, baby girl. After a few years of enjoying time with their little miracle, they realized they wanted a sibling for their only child. Considering they had no remaining embryos from the first cycle, and still needed intervention to get pregnant, they decided to do IVF again, but this time at a clinic in Chicago. In February 2016, they transferred two very good quality embryos but did not get pregnant. Although they were distraught about the failed cycle, they were still grateful for their daughter and thankful they still had four frozen embryos to try again when ready.

When they were ready to try again, they found out the four frozen embryos were not viable and, after spending thousands of dollars more at this clinic, they were once again back to square one. After depleting their resources and still not having another baby, Gina decided to look into other options to make her dream come true. She decided to pick up a part-time job at Starbucks for four months, on top of her full-time teaching position, to get fertility coverage. It worked! After getting the coverage, she was able to get another laparoscopic surgery in August 2016 and then began IVF #3 in October 2016 at Aurora in Wisconsin. They made a few modifications to her protocol, and she ended up with three embryos. They decided to send the embryos off for genetic testing, prior to transferring, for the best possible chance of success, considering Gina had some known issues in this area. Out of the three embryos, one was considered genetically normal. They transferred that one in February of 2017 and had a second beautiful, baby girl!

Note: If you are considering traveling abroad for IVF, Gina speaks highly of their clinic, so I thought I'd provide information if you would like to look into Gennet further: https://www.gennet.cz/en/

Story # 2: I will do whatever it takes to become a mom.

Em was in her early thirties when she and her husband began trying to start their family. After trying Clomid cycles and other hormone injections for three and a half years with no success, and having a miscarriage, the next step was IVF. At this time, the only issue she knew was preventing her from conception was the fact that she did not ovulate on her own. Therefore, Em and her husband knew for sure that IVF would allow them to have a baby. Although they were right, it definitely did not happen the way they expected. It took them four years to bring a baby home.

Em did her first IVF cycle and ended up with twenty usable embryos! She had a total of eight FET transfers from this batch and still did not have a baby.

- At least six of the embryos transferred had been tested PGS normal. The rest were not tested.
- Of the eight transfers, Em got pregnant four times and she miscarried all four within the fifth week of pregnancy.

After these last eight failed attempts, four which resulted in implantation, Em and her husband figured the issue may not be with the embryos, but rather with Em's body's ability to sustain a pregnancy. Being out of embryos, back to square one, and still determined to have a baby, they made the difficult decision to do a second IVF cycle, but this time use a gestational carrier. Having another IVF cycle meant there would be another egg retrieval, but they were ready. After producing twenty transferable embryos the first time, they thought for sure there would be just as many this time. However, this cycle ONLY yielded one embryo, so they decided not to do PGS testing and took their chances and transferred to their gestational carrier. That one embryo implanted and resulted in their beautiful son who they named Nathan, meaning "gift from God."

While their gestational carrier was pregnant with their baby, Em did a third IVF egg retrieval to get more embryos for future children. They now have three frozen embryos that were PGS normal based on the genetic testing. After having additional testing on herself, she believes they may have found the root cause of the recurrent miscarriages and, with a new, very specialized protocol, she will be trying a transfer to her own uterus in the future.

Story #3: I will not allow negative news to cause me to abort my dream of becoming a mom.

Darryl and Mikka tried for several years to have a baby together. They got pregnant several times during those years, but either had a miscarriage or an ectopic each time. Finally, Mikka had to get one of her fallopian tubes removed, leaving her with just the remaining one, which was blocked. Left with no way to conceive naturally, IVF was the next step.

Preparing Your Perspective

They came up with the money, scheduled their consultation appointment, and then proceeded with the procedure. Three of their embryos made it to day three, so because of age (she was thirty-nine) and other factors, the doctor decided to transfer all of them into Mikka's uterus. She and her husband waited patiently for the pregnancy test and, just as suspected, they were indeed pregnant. A few weeks later, they had their very first ultrasound. To their surprise, two of the three embryos had implanted. They were having twins!

As time, progressed, they found out that they were not only having twins, but boy/girl twins. How cute! As the second trimester was almost coming to a close, and the third trimester was being ushered in, they were once again surprised. This time, the surprise called for some serious prayer and strong faith. Mikka went into labor at twenty-five weeks. The doctors told her and her husband that the babies had fluid on their brains and would possibly be MRDD, so they suggested terminating the pregnancy. After praying and believing, they decided not to go with that option, but rather to believe God and give birth to the twins at twenty-five weeks. One was 1 lb. 9 oz, and the other was 1 lb. 13 oz. The umbilical cord cut off their oxygen at birth, one needed resuscitation, and they both had low birth weight. The babies were not expected to survive, but after a heart surgery at one month old, developmental delays, and even hearing loss, both babies are now doing wonderful. They are now five years old, functioning in school with no delays, and beating the odds!

Story #4: It only takes one good embryo to have a healthy baby.

Jessica and her husband tried for years to have a child. After seven miscarriages, she found out that she had a genetic disorder which may result in her babies having Trisomy 22, which is incompatible with life and causes first trimester loss if present. They were told that the only way to ensure their pregnancy lasts was to do IVF with PGS testing, so they could only transfer genetically normal embryos. Jessica and her husband were very hopeful, because they knew they did not have an issue getting pregnant. The issue was with staying pregnant. They proceeded with IVF and sent the seven embryos that made it to day five for testing. Of those seven, only one was considered "normal," meaning neither Trisomy 22 nor any other genetic issue was detected. They transferred that embryo, survived the two-week wait, and then did a pregnancy test. The result was negative. Jessica and her husband were devastated because their only normal embryo did not implant, and they did not have any more money to try IVF again.

Two months later, Jessica found out she was pregnant naturally. She was afraid to get excited because of her history with genetic issues. Each week she waited to miscarry, until finally one day, she was in the second trimester, further in pregnancy than she had ever made it in the past. Jessica carried this baby full-term and had a healthy baby boy, naturally, despite the odds.

꩜ Journal ꩜

When there is a problem, do you usually see the glass half full or half empty?

Do you think you have the proper perspective to become a mom against all odds?

Do you personally know anyone who has struggled with infertility and then had a baby?

Part III
PURSUING

Chapter 7

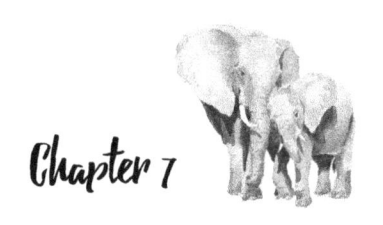

DON'T FORGET THAT HE WILL BE A DAD

One of my favorite movies of all time is *The Lion King*. I know it's a "kids" movie, but guess what; I love kids movies. I don't know how many times I've watched the movie, but I do know that I can quote the majority of the lines and all of the song lyrics. The story is about a little lion, Simba, who was destined to be king. At first Simba was excited and could not wait to be king. Then his father, King Mufasa, was killed and his Uncle Scar (Mufasa's brother) convinced him that it was all his fault. This caused Simba to run away from home as a child. He left his mother, other family members, and best friend Nala, and went to a faraway land where he could hide from his calling to be king, even though he once couldn't wait for it. He grew up, became an adult, and then he ran back into Nala while roaming around in the wilderness. Although he saw himself as a grown-up lion, when she saw him, she saw him as the king, the highest authority in the jungle. She didn't know why he had run away all those years ago, or what he was hiding from. All she knew was that he did not see himself the way she saw him. She eventually helped him rediscover his full potential, face his fears, and return home to take his place as king!

Going through this infertility journey, I discovered that my husband was a lot like Simba. For a time, he was hiding the fact that he really wanted to be a father because he was afraid that he wouldn't be a "good" one. He could not see himself being a dad because he was not raised by his. After he opened up to me about these feelings, I was able to encourage him by expressing that I can tell he will be a good father by how he takes care of me and handles all of his responsibilities. I assured him that I have no doubt about it. I saw him as the highest authority in our home, a father, and my husband, and I made sure he knew it. Once he got over that hurdle, we had various other hurdles in our journey. Just when we started to get excited, we would get another let-down. We were on an emotional rollercoaster, but at least we were together. I knew how I felt, but I wondered what he was thinking. Even though I saw him break down and cry a few times during our losses, he demonstrated such strength and unshakable faith, which comforted me and provided stability when my feelings wavered. I learned that as you pursue motherhood, you can't forget that while you will be a mom, your man will be a dad. Therefore, you can't discount his feelings or forget that he is also going through this journey as well. I taught myself to not get easily offended by him during this time, because men express emotions differently than women. It is vitally important that you understand this and work with your man, not against him, as you pursue parenthood together.

> Work with your man, not against him, as you pursue parenthood together.

Here are ways you can strengthen your union during these challenging times:

- Communicate with each other about your feelings.
- Compliment him for things he is doing well.

- Try not to nag about little things.
- Choose your battles. Everything is not worth creating drama over.
- Take a vacation or weekend getaway.
- Have sex when he wants it. This will help him relieve stress.
- Surprise him by getting dressed up for him and making him a nice dinner.
- Give him space to enjoy the activities he loves when he needs it.

In an effort to help take a look into the mind of a man, I asked my husband questions about our journey from his perspective and I thought I'd share his responses with you:

1. **My question:** When we first started trying to conceive, what made you most afraid about being a dad?

His answer: He thought he wasn't going to be a good father because he was not raised by his father.

2. **My question**: What did I do or say during this journey to conceiving that got on your nerves or made you feel pressured?

His answer: The only pressure he felt was the financial pressure. He was wondering how we were going to handle living expenses, unexpected house/car repairs, save money, and pay for IVF.

3. **My question**: What were your thoughts/feelings when you discovered that we were going to need intervention to get pregnant?

His answer: He was initially worried. He wondered about the following:

- How we were going to get the money?
- What he was going to be responsible for during the procedure?
- Were we going to need a surrogate?
- Was my body capable of having a baby?
- If I already had problems getting pregnant, did that mean I was going to have problems in my pregnancy?
- Does the procedure actually work?
- Are the success rates accurate, or do doctors inflate them just to make more money?
- What if we did it and it didn't work?

4. **My question:** How do you think this journey has affected our marriage?

His answer: He said it brought us closer together. He mentioned that he reflected on our marriage vows and realized this process revealed that he really was with me in "sickness and in health." He learned that he can be a caretaker. Prior to going through this process he was scared of needles, but he ended up giving me all the necessary shots for the procedures. He said he thought he couldn't do it at first, but he found a way to push past his discomfort because of his love for me and our future child.

5. **My question:** What changed your perspective about being a dad and got you more excited about it?

His answer: The idea of being a dad gave him something to look forward to that is beyond him. He was also inspired by seeing how happy his friends, men in the church, and coworkers are to be fathers. They made fatherhood look attractive. He imagined himself being a father and felt life would be more exciting and have more meaning. He wondered:

- Who is the baby going to be?
- What will the baby look like? Whose features will he or she have?
- What types of activities will he do with our child?

6. My question: Did you learn anything new about your wife or yourself while going through this journey?

His answer: Yes. Seeing me go through all the stuff I had to go through showed him that I'm willing to go through whatever is necessary to have our child. He appreciated my strength and had to learn to support me in different ways. Even though he provides for me and takes care of me, he felt helpless during parts of this journey. He used the analogy that he fixes computers and solves IT issues daily. He takes that approach in every problem, but it was frustrating not being about to solve our infertility problem and just take the pain away from me. Not being able to alleviate the issue taught him that he needed to learn to be there for me emotionally.

7. My question: Do you feel going through this process made you and your wife closer?

His answer: Yes.

Talking to him reminded me that he had some of the same thoughts and fears that I had, and even though he did not always express those thoughts and feelings, they were there. I appreciate his transparency and partnership during our journey.

As you pursue being a mom, look at your man and remember, he WILL be a dad!

Journal

During this journey, have you considered your husband's feelings? Explain.

What have you learned about you or your husband so far while going through this process?

Which of your husband's qualities are you most thankful for?

Chapter 8

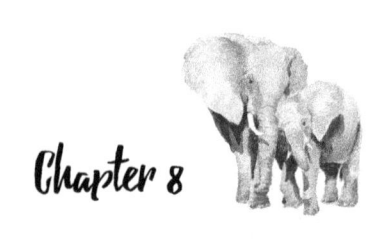

IT'S TIME TO PUSH!

It is time to PUSH! Yes, ladies; you read it correctly. It is time to PUSH! After the labor pains, proper dilation, and effacement, the baby is finally ready to be delivered. However, it will take some pushing to get there. By this stage, the most difficult parts are usually over, and you just have to help guide your baby out of the birth canal to experience the moment you have been waiting for the entire pregnancy: holding your baby. For those of us who have struggled with infertility, there are also pre-labor pains that happen even before pregnancy. In your infertility journey, there are pains, uncomfortable experiences, tears, and even unexpected hurdles to go through: all to get to the moment you have been waiting for, pregnancy. During this process, you will have to push past many obstacles, but as long as you are informed about them in advance, you will know how to take deep breaths and "push" until you get what you want.

Pushing Through Financial Barriers

Paying for infertility treatments is not cheap. While some women have endless resources or benefits to pay for all of the treatments and medications needed to achieve motherhood, some of us don't. There are also circumstances where you had enough to start the journey, but ended up with unexpected costs. Regardless of your situation, in this section, I will provide tips on how my husband and I were able to pay for three full IVF cycles and one FET cycle, including all medications. Each IVF cycle at the clinic I went to was a little over $7,043 and the medications for each cycle ranged from $5,000 to about $6,500, depending on the protocol. The FET cycle was about $3,400, including the medications. It cost us over $45,000 to bring our first baby home. This does not include the surgeries, Clomid cycles, additional testing, or other miscellaneous fees. The financial barrier was definitely one of the toughest barriers to get through.

> People find money to do the things they really want to do.

I didn't expect to have to go through so much for one baby, but I quickly realized that people find money to do the things they really want to do. Even though we started off with a budget and a plan, the costs kept increasing as the journey got longer. We had to get very creative with ways to either pay or come up with additional money. We did and I am happy to say that it was all worth it, and if I had to do it all over again, I would.

When we first found out how much we were going to need to do our first IVF cycle, we wondered how we would come up with the money; but since we really wanted to have a baby, we decided that we would find a way. Here are the various methods my husband and I used to fund our future baby:

- Went through closets and sold some of my old clothes and shoes that were in good condition to consignments shops or using various selling apps.
- Created a Gofundme page and asked various friends and family to contribute. I will admit this was one of

the hardest ones for me to do because I have never liked to ask anyone for anything or share my story, because I felt it was too personal.
- On my thirty-second birthday, I had a small get-together at my house and asked friends and family that could to each give me $32.
- Purchased Anthony Thomas© candy bars and one of my cousins sold them at her job for me.
- Shared our story with friends and family and, occasionally, people would just give us a contribution towards it.
- Worked at Starbucks part-time until I was able to get benefits.
- Maintained the Starbucks benefits through COBRA after quitting.
- Buying furniture and other home goods from online auctions and selling those items on various selling apps.
- I even signed up to be an Uber driver, but decided not to because hubby didn't like the idea.
- Saved extra money from our paychecks by cutting excess spending. For a time, we did not buy any fast food or take any trips to save as much money as possible.
- Used credit cards when necessary.
- I looked into borrowing money from my 401k, but decided against it because I really didn't want to do it unless it was absolutely necessary.
- Asked clinic if anyone had donated extra medications that I could have.
- Communicated on infertility forums regularly. Because several ladies were familiar with my story, one of my infertility friend warriors, Gina, sent me a few boxes of Menopur and progesterone, which came in handy.

Another lady offered me some of her leftover meds, but since they were not the ones that were a part of my protocol, I could not accept them. However, the fact that these ladies thought of me after they finished their cycles and had their babies really warmed my heart.
- Applied for the Companionate Care program to get discounts on medications.
- Started a store on Etsy selling T-shirts and socks.

Here are some other ways to come up with the money that we researched, but didn't use:

- Take out a loan.
- Apply for infertility grant programs.
- Switch clinics to one that is less expensive.
- Get treatment overseas.
- Find a clinic that has a shared risk program. (You get a partial refund if you don't get a baby after a certain number of cycles.)
- Look into switching your health insurance to have a flexible spending account with a HSA, if that is an option at your company.
- Adopt an embryo.
- See if you are a good candidate for mini-IVF.

Now, it's time for you to evaluate your own financial situation and think about how you will fund your miracle baby. After you find out the estimated cost of your treatment, answer the following questions:

1. How much money will you be able to save each month?

2. What are some unnecessary expenses you can cut out to prioritize this process?

3. How soon do you think you will be able to start or continue the process?

4. How many rounds of fertility treatments do you think you will be able to afford before having to quit?

5. After paying for fertility treatments, will you still have money saved in case of an emergency?

6. What creative methods can you use to bring in additional income?

7. Do you have any relatives or friends that would help you? If so, who are they?

_____

_____

_____

_____

_____

Pushing Through All of the Appointments

During this journey you will likely have a lot of doctor's appointments, testing to complete, and medications to take. This can be physically and emotionally draining. However, keep your eyes on the prize and document next steps so you don't miss anything. Even though you are pushing through these appointments, there are important details you don't want to miss.

Tips for Keeping Track of it All

- Research your clinic's SART scores to determine their success rate.
- Mark all scheduled appointments on your calendar.
- If your doctor gave you a protocol calendar with medications and dates to start them, print it out and place it somewhere visible to you. Look at it daily.
- Ask any questions about medications during your appointments, or call the nurse line if you think of something later.

- Keep track of your next steps using an infertility app.
- If you have a failed cycle or a result that you were not expecting, be sure to write down questions in advance to ask the doctor.
- Always take all medications the doctor gives you in the prescribed dosages at the correct time.
- Arrive to all appointments on time. Usually when getting fertility treatments, timing is important.
- If you feel you are not receiving the care you need, get a second opinion.
- See a counselor if necessary to determine if you are emotionally ready to continue the journey.
- Do research on your unique situation, so you have a better understanding of what you may need to discuss with your doctor.

Upcoming Appointments

1. When is your next appointment?

_____

_____

_____

_____

_____

2. Do you know what questions you will ask your doctor at your next appointment? If not, you should write them down and bring them so you don't forget.

3. Is there anything you want to share with your doctor? If so, what is it?

_____

_____

_____

_____

_____

_____

There were a few appointments that were very emotional for me that I really needed to push through:

- First consultation for IVF – I was nervous because I didn't know what to expect.
- Follow-up appointments after a loss – Pulling up to the building brought back all of the memories and emotions surrounding the loss.
- Follow-up appointments after a failed cycle — Pulling up to the building brought back all of the memories and emotions surrounding everything I went through, only to have a failed cycle.

Even though some of your appointments may bring back memories or make you feel emotional, push past those feelings and realize the appointment is getting you one step closer to your baby.

Pushing Through in Prayer

Many years ago, I was at a church service and there was a speaker there who preached a message called PUSH: Pray until Something Happens. As I was going through this journey, this message came to my remembrance because the analogies that were used to get the point across surrounded childbirth. I realized that after all I had been through to get pregnant, I was not in control and I could not make it happen. I had to do my part but also walk in faith. This caused me to increase my prayer life to ensure I believed that God was able to make it happen.

Prayer definitely helped my husband and I get through my journey, so if you are someone who prays, I would encourage you to do exactly as we did, pray until something happens. I have heard that if you do anything for twenty-one days, it becomes a habit or part of your lifestyle. Therefore, I have added some prayers that you can pray every day for thirty days. Once the month is up, feel free to start the prayers over again or make up your own daily prayers.

Thirty Days of PUSHing

Day 1

Scripture: "Now indeed, Elizabeth your relative has also conceived a son in her old age; and this is now the sixth month for her who was called barren. For with God nothing will be impossible" (Luke 1:36-37, NKJV).

Prayer: Dear Lord, I know there is still hope for me to have a baby. My age doesn't matter and neither does any physical limitations I am facing. There is NOTHING that is impossible for You! I am not the first woman to battle infertility, and I am sure I won't be the last. I know that since You were able to help many other woman have their rainbow babies, I know that it is still possible for me to have mine as well. Thank you in advance for making my dream of becoming a mom come to pass.

Thoughts After Today's Prayer

_____

_____

_____

_____

_____

_____

_____

_____

Day 2

Scripture: "Hear me when I call, O God of my righteousness! You have relieved me in my distress;
Have mercy on me, and hear my prayer" (Psalm 4:1, NKJV).

Prayer: Dear Lord, You know my heart and You are aware of all I have been through up to this point. I know that You have given me the strength to continue pursuing my dream, so I ask that You continue to hear my prayers and comfort me in the times of distress. Your word tells me to ask and I will receive. I am asking You to allow me the opportunity to complete my family with a baby. Thank you in advance for making my dream of becoming a mom come to pass.

Thoughts After Today's Prayer

Day 3

Scripture: "For which of you, intending to build a tower, does not sit down first and count the cost, whether he has enough to finish it— lest, after he has laid the foundation, and is not able to finish, all who see it begin to mock him, saying, 'This man began to build and was not able to finish'" (Luke 14:28-30, NKJV).

Prayer: Dear Lord, as I prepare to become a mom, I thank you for reminding me to count the cost before building my family. I understand that my life is going to change, and I am prepared for this change. I thank you that I will do my part and rely on You for the rest. I know You will supply all of our needs so I am not worried about not having enough. My family is built on the foundation of faith and belief that You are able to do anything!

Thoughts After Today's Prayer

_____

_____

_____

_____

_____

_____

_____

_____

Day 4

Scripture: "Rejoice always, pray without ceasing, in everything give thanks; for this is the will of God in Christ Jesus for you" (1 Thessalonians 5:16-18, NKJV).

Prayer: Dear Lord, help me not to be so consumed with this journey and what is going wrong that I lose sight of all the things that are going right. I will rejoice always and be glad. Help me to remain thankful for even the little things. I don't want to take anything for granted. I will continue to pray until something happens! Thank you in advance for making my dream of becoming a mom come to pass.

Thoughts After Today's Prayer

Day 5

Scripture: "To everything there is a season,
A time for every purpose under heaven:
A time to be born,
And a time to die;
A time to plant,
And a time to pluck what is planted;" (Ecclesiastes 3:1-2, NKJV).

Prayer: Dear Lord, I realize there is a time for everything. I don't know when I will have my baby, but I do know I will. Therefore, I will keep moving forward and doing what I can until it's my turn. Thank you in advance for making my dream of becoming a mom come to pass.

Thoughts After Today's Prayer

Day 6

Scripture: "For we are glad when we are weak and you are strong. And this also we pray, that you may be made complete" (2 Corinthians 13:9, NKJV).

Prayer: Dear Lord, at times I get weak during this journey, but I am thankful that when I am weak, You are still strong. You are more than capable of opening my womb and causing me to be able to not only conceive, but to carry my baby to term as well. Thank you in advance for making my dream of becoming a mom come to pass.

Thoughts After Today's Prayer

Day 7

Scripture: "Ah, Lord God! Behold, You have made the heavens and the earth by Your great power and outstretched arm. There is nothing too hard for You" (Jeremiah 32:17, NKJV).

Prayer: Dear Lord, today I just want to thank You because there is nothing too hard for You. Thank you in advance for making my dream of becoming a mom come to pass.

Thoughts After Today's Prayer

Day 8

Scripture: "She makes linen garments and sells them,
And supplies sashes for the merchants.
Strength and honor are her clothing;
She shall rejoice in time to come" (Proverbs 31:24-25, NKJV).

Prayer: Dear Lord, help me to be a virtuous woman no matter what my situation is. Help me to use the gifts and talents You have given me to produce more resources for my household. There are a lot of unknown expenses that pop up during this infertility journey. Bless me with enough to handle all of them. I thank You for always being a provider, and even though I don't always know how the provision will be made, I know You always make a way.

Thoughts After Today's Prayer

Day 9

Scripture: "But He said, 'The things which are impossible with men are possible with God'" (Luke 18:27, NKJV).

Prayer: Dear Lord, today I just want to thank You because there is nothing too hard for You. I know that the doctors can't make me get pregnant and neither can I. I am not in control; You are. Thank you in advance for making my dream of becoming a mom come to pass.

Thoughts After Today's Prayer

Day 10

Scripture: "I have set the Lord always before me; Because He is at my right hand I shall not be moved" (Psalm 16:8, NKJV).

Prayer: Dear Lord, even though this journey has not been as easy as I'd hoped it would be, help me to stand firm on my faith and not be moved. I know that You are with me, and You can sustain me by Your power.

Thoughts After Today's Prayer

Day 11

Scripture: "And not being weak in faith, he did not consider his own body, already dead (since he was about a hundred years old), and the deadness of Sarah's womb." (Romans 4:19, NKJV).

Prayer: Dear Lord, at times my faith gets weak, but I know when I am weak You are strong. Help me not to focus on my surroundings, weaknesses, or physical limitations. Even though it seems as if at times there is no hope, I recognize that there is nothing too hard for You, and You don't need a perfect situation to make a situation perfect.

> You don't need a perfect situation to make a situation perfect.

Thoughts After Today's Prayer

Day 12

Scripture: "He did not waver at the promise of God through unbelief, but was strengthened in faith, giving glory to God" (Romans 4:20, NKJV).

Prayer: Dear Lord, I give You all the glory, honor, and praise. I know You are well able to give me the opportunity to be a mom and to have the baby that I have been desiring. Help me not to waver, but to stay focused on the promise.

Thoughts After Today's Prayer

Day 13

Scripture: "and being fully convinced that what He had promised He was also able to perform" (Romans 4:21, NKJV).

Prayer: Dear Lord, I am convinced that You can do it. There is no doubt in my mind. I know I will have my baby soon, and I am so grateful for Your reassurance.

Thoughts After Today's Prayer

Day 14

Scripture: "And not only that, but we also glory in tribulations, knowing that tribulation produces perseverance; and perseverance, character; and character, hope" (Romans 5:3-4, NKJV).

Prayer: Dear Lord, although I do not like that I have had to wait longer than I wanted to and have a tougher time getting pregnant than I anticipated, I am thankful to know that I am much stronger than I thought I was. This journey has shown me that I have the tenacity to persevere through any obstacle to get what I want. I have changed so much for the better during this journey and have learned to deal with various emotions, and still manage to believe that I will still get to be a mom. I have not lost my hope, and I will continue to pursue my dream until my baby is in my arms. Even though I have wanted to get out of the journey, I am thankful that You are getting me through it.

Thoughts After Today's Prayer

Day 15

Scripture: "Therefore, having been justified by faith, we have peace with God through our Lord Jesus Christ" (Romans 5:1, NKJV).

Prayer: Dear Lord, I thank you for peace that passes all understanding. I may not have all the answers, but I have You. Please continue to give me peace. I let go of worry and pick up trust. I trust You will help my dream of being a mom come to pass.

Thoughts After Today's Prayer

Day 16

Scripture: "Rejoice with those who rejoice, and weep with those who weep" (Romans 12:15, NKJV).

Prayer: Dear Lord, I recognize that everyone around me may not understand what I am going through and may not be sensitive to my feelings. Help me to rejoice when others get pregnant and not be envious, jealous, or sad because it isn't my turn yet. Help me to still be able to empathize with others who may be struggling to become mothers as well, even once I have my baby. I praise You in advance for what You are doing in my life, and I will rejoice and be glad because I know it will happen for me.

Thoughts After Today's Prayer

Day 17

Scripture: "Be kindly affectionate to one another with brotherly love, in honor giving preference to one another;" (Romans 12:10, NKJV).

Prayer: Dear Lord, help me not to be so consumed with my own issues that I neglect those around me and become desensitized to the feelings of others. I am confident that You are able to bless me with a child, so I can manage my emotions and choose to be happy.

Thoughts After Today's Prayer

Day 18

Scripture: "For God has not given us a spirit of fear, but of power and of love and of a sound mind" (2 Timothy 1:7, NKJV).

Prayer: Dear Lord, I thank you for a sound mind that is free from anxiety, worry, or fear. You have not given me a reason to fear or fret, so today I will choose to focus on the positive and be hopeful in all situations.

Thoughts After Today's Prayer

Day 19

Scripture: "And take the helmet of salvation, and the sword of the Spirit, which is the word of God;" (Ephesians 6:17, NKJV).

Prayer: Dear Lord, help me to guard my mind from all negativity. I don't want to listen to or focus on anything that will distract me, cause me to lose my faith, or makes me waiver in my beliefs. I will use positive affirmations and Your word to combat any negative thought. Surround me with people who encourage and give me hope.

Thoughts After Today's Prayer

Day 20

Scripture: "being confident of this very thing, that He who has begun a good work in you will complete it until the day of Jesus Christ;" (Philippians 1:6, NKJV).

Prayer: Dear Lord, it's not over until it's over! I started this journey with You and I am confident that You will complete the work that was started. I am adding works to my faith, and I know that You will do the rest. I thank you that I will be a mom.

Thoughts After Today's Prayer

Day 21

Scripture: "Brethren, I do not count myself to have apprehended; but one thing I do, forgetting those things which are behind and reaching forward to those things which are ahead" (Philippians 3:13, NKJV).

Prayer: Dear Lord, I have had failures and disappointments in the past, but help me to forget those and look forward to all of the great things that are ahead of me. I realize that my past does not dictate my future, but rather prepares me for it. This journey has prepared me to be a good mom, so when I get discouraged I will choose to focus on that.

Thoughts After Today's Prayer

Day 22

Scripture: "I press toward the goal for the prize of the upward call of God in Christ Jesus" (Philippians 3:14, NKJV).

Prayer: Dear Lord, thank you for giving me the strength to keep going, even when I wanted to quit. I know I will not regret it when I am holding my baby in my arms. I will keep pushing forward until I reach my goal.

Thoughts After Today's Prayer

Day 23

Scripture: "Brethren, join in following my example, and note those who so walk, as you have us for a pattern" (Philippians 3:17, NKJV).

Prayer: Dear Lord, I realize that there are so many other women who struggle with infertility. Allow me to be exposed to women that have had similar struggles and still had a baby so I am reminded that it is possible. Also, help me to go through this journey in such a way that other woman struggling to get pregnant are encouraged to keep pursuing their dreams as well.

Thoughts After Today's Prayer

Day 24

Scripture: "Rejoice in the Lord always. Again I will say, rejoice!" (Philippians 4:4, NKJV).

Prayer: Dear Lord, I will rejoice and be glad. Despite what happens, I will be happy. You are still good! At times situations and circumstances attempt to steal my joy, but I know that You are in control, so I will maintain my joy and choose to believe that everything will work out for me. Thank you for guarding my mind and helping me focus on the positive in every situation.

Thoughts After Today's Prayer

Day 25

Scripture: "Be anxious for nothing, but in everything by prayer and supplication, with thanksgiving, let your requests be made known to God;" (Philippians 4:6, NKJV).

Prayer: Dear Lord, help me not to be anxious, but to remain prayerful. Sometimes I get worried, but I know that I have no reason to worry. You are in control, so I will do my part and let You do Yours. I thank you for all You have done for me and I appreciate Your faithfulness. Thank you for guarding my mind and giving me peace that passes all understanding.

Thoughts After Today's Prayer

Day 26

Scripture: "and the peace of God, which surpasses all understanding, will guard your hearts and minds through Christ Jesus" (Philippians 4:7, NKJV).

Prayer: Dear Lord, You are in control, so I will do my part and let You do Yours. I thank you for all You have done for me, and I appreciate Your faithfulness. Thank you for guarding my mind and giving me peace that passes all understanding.

Thoughts After Today's Prayer

Day 27

Scripture: "Finally, brethren, whatever things are true, whatever things are noble, whatever things are just, whatever things are pure, whatever things are lovely, whatever things are of good report, if there is any virtue and if there is anything praiseworthy—meditate on these things" (Philippians 4:8, NKJV).

Prayer: Dear Lord, help me to maintain a positive outlook. Help me to focus on the truth of Your word, good news, and doing the right thing, even if I don't see the desired result as quickly as I wanted. I am going to praise You in advance because I know that You will bless me with the child I desire.

Thoughts After Today's Prayer

Day 28

Scripture: "I know how to be abased, and I know how to abound. Everywhere and in all things I have learned both to be full and to be hungry, both to abound and to suffer need" (Philippians 4:12, NKJV).

Prayer: Dear Lord, thank you for teaching me to be content in all things. Although I am still waiting on my promise, I will be grateful for where I am and the blessings I already have. I am going to praise You in advance, because I know that You will bless me with the child I desire.

Thoughts After Today's Prayer

_____
_____
_____
_____
_____
_____
_____
_____
_____
_____
_____

Day 29

Scripture: "I can do all things through Christ who strengthens me" (Philippians 4:13, NKJV).

Prayer: Dear Lord, although sometimes I feel like giving up and feel like I won't be able to take anymore, I realize that with Your help I can do anything as You strengthen me. Thank you for keeping me and giving me joy, despite the difficulties in my life. You deserve the glory, the honor, and the praise. Thank you for all You do.

Thoughts After Today's Prayer

Day 30

Scripture: "For this child I prayed, and the Lord has granted me my petition which I asked of Him. Therefore I also have lent him to the Lord; as long as he lives he shall be lent to the Lord." So they worshiped the Lord there" (1 Samuel 1:27-28, NKJV).

Prayer: Dear Lord, I thank you in advance for blessing me with the child that I have been praying for. I thank you for allowing me to have the endurance to keep going, even when I wanted to quit. Thank you for being a provider and a keeper. I will dedicate this child to You, and teach my child to pray and to serve You as well. You are a great God, an awesome God, the only God. You deserve all the glory, honor, and praise.

Thoughts After Today's Prayer

Chapter 9

TRACKING YOUR PURSUIT

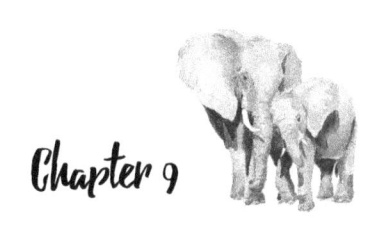

Tracking your pursuit by journaling can be very important to your emotional growth because it is therapeutic. It shows your progress in chronological order and allows you to look back and be reminded of important milestones from your journey. Use this chapter to document your journey to becoming a mom. If you need more space, feel free to use a separate notebook to capture these memories using the same template.

Before you get started with the daily journal, write a letter to your future self, as if you have already won the battle against infertility and completed your family. Consider what you have learned along the journey, how you'll feel when you are holding your child for the first time, and what your life is like at that point. Once you have your child, read this letter again.

Letter to Your Future Self

Date _____

Dear _____ ,

Daily Journal – Tracking Your Pursuit

Day 1

What was your mood today?

    a) Happy
    b) Sad
    c) Angry
    d) Other

Why did you feel this way?

_____

_____

_____

_____

_____

What are you most thankful for today?

_____

_____

_____

_____

_____

Did you achieve your goals for the day? Why or why not?

Daily Journal Entry

Tracking Your Pursuit

Day 2

What was your mood today?

- a) Happy
- b) Sad
- c) Angry
- d) Other

Why did you feel this way?

_____

_____

_____

_____

_____

_____

What are you most thankful for today?

_____

_____

_____

_____

_____

_____

Tracking Your Pursuit

Did you achieve your goals for the day? Why or why not?

Daily Journal Entry

I STILL Want To Be A Mom

Day 3

What was your mood today?

    a) Happy
    b) Sad
    c) Angry
    d) Other

Why did you feel this way?

What are you most thankful for today?

Did you achieve your goals for the day? Why or why not?

Daily Journal Entry

Tracking Your Pursuit

Day 4

What was your mood today?

    a) Happy
    b) Sad
    c) Angry
    d) Other

Why did you feel this way?

_____

_____

_____

_____

_____

_____

What are you most thankful for today?

_____

_____

_____

_____

_____

_____

Tracking Your Pursuit

Did you achieve your goals for the day? Why or why not?

___

Daily Journal Entry

___

I STILL Want To Be A Mom

Day 5

What was your mood today?

    a) Happy
    b) Sad
    c) Angry
    d) Other

Why did you feel this way?

_____
_____
_____
_____
_____

What are you most thankful for today?

_____
_____
_____
_____
_____

Did you achieve your goals for the day? Why or why not?

Daily Journal Entry

Tracking Your Pursuit

Day 6

What was your mood today?

    a) Happy
    b) Sad
    c) Angry
    d) Other

Why did you feel this way?

_____

_____

_____

_____

_____

What are you most thankful for today?

_____

_____

_____

_____

_____

_____

_____

Did you achieve your goals for the day? Why or why not?

Daily Journal Entry

I STILL Want To Be A Mom

Day 7

What was your mood today?

    a) Happy
    b) Sad
    c) Angry
    d) Other

Why did you feel this way?

_____

_____

_____

_____

_____

What are you most thankful for today?

_____

_____

_____

_____

_____

_____

I STILL Want To Be A Mom

Did you achieve your goals for the day? Why or why not?

Daily Journal Entry

Tracking Your Pursuit

Day 8

What was your mood today?

- a) Happy
- b) Sad
- c) Angry
- d) Other

Why did you feel this way?

_____
_____
_____
_____
_____

What are you most thankful for today?

_____
_____
_____
_____
_____
_____
_____

Tracking Your Pursuit

Did you achieve your goals for the day? Why or why not?

Daily Journal Entry

I STILL Want To Be A Mom

Day 9

What was your mood today?

    a) Happy
    b) Sad
    c) Angry
    d) Other

Why did you feel this way?

What are you most thankful for today?

I STILL Want To Be A Mom

Did you achieve your goals for the day? Why or why not?

_____

_____

_____

_____

_____

_____

Daily Journal Entry

_____

_____

_____

_____

_____

_____

_____

_____

_____

_____

_____

_____

Tracking Your Pursuit

Day 10

What was your mood today?

- a) Happy
- b) Sad
- c) Angry
- d) Other

Why did you feel this way?

_____
_____
_____
_____
_____

What are you most thankful for today?

_____
_____
_____
_____
_____
_____
_____

Tracking Your Pursuit

Did you achieve your goals for the day? Why or why not?

Daily Journal Entry

I STILL Want To Be A Mom

Day 11

What was your mood today?

   a) Happy
   b) Sad
   c) Angry
   d) Other

Why did you feel this way?

_____

_____

_____

_____

_____

_____

What are you most thankful for today?

_____

_____

_____

_____

_____

_____

I STILL Want To Be A Mom

Did you achieve your goals for the day? Why or why not?

_____

_____

_____

_____

_____

_____

Daily Journal Entry

_____

_____

_____

_____

_____

_____

_____

_____

_____

_____

_____

_____

Tracking Your Pursuit

Day 12

What was your mood today?

    a) Happy
    b) Sad
    c) Angry
    d) Other

Why did you feel this way?

What are you most thankful for today?

Did you achieve your goals for the day? Why or why not?

Daily Journal Entry

I STILL Want To Be A Mom

Day 13

What was your mood today?

   a) Happy
   b) Sad
   c) Angry
   d) Other

Why did you feel this way?

_____

_____

_____

_____

_____

_____

What are you most thankful for today?

_____

_____

_____

_____

_____

_____

Did you achieve your goals for the day? Why or why not?

Daily Journal Entry

Tracking Your Pursuit

Day 14

What was your mood today?

    a) Happy
    b) Sad
    c) Angry
    d) Other

Why did you feel this way?

_____
_____
_____
_____
_____
_____

What are you most thankful for today?

_____
_____
_____
_____
_____
_____

Tracking Your Pursuit

Did you achieve your goals for the day? Why or why not?

Daily Journal Entry

I STILL Want To Be A Mom

Day 15

What was your mood today?

    a) Happy
    b) Sad
    c) Angry
    d) Other

Why did you feel this way?

What are you most thankful for today?

I STILL Want To Be A Mom

Did you achieve your goals for the day? Why or why not?

Daily Journal Entry

Tracking Your Pursuit

Day 16

What was your mood today?

    a) Happy
    b) Sad
    c) Angry
    d) Other

Why did you feel this way?

_____
_____
_____
_____
_____
_____

What are you most thankful for today?

_____
_____
_____
_____
_____
_____
_____

Did you achieve your goals for the day? Why or why not?

Daily Journal Entry

I STILL Want To Be A Mom

Day 17

What was your mood today?

- a) Happy
- b) Sad
- c) Angry
- d) Other

Why did you feel this way?

___

What are you most thankful for today?

___

I STILL Want To Be A Mom

Did you achieve your goals for the day? Why or why not?

_____

_____

_____

_____

_____

_____

Daily Journal Entry

_____

_____

_____

_____

_____

_____

_____

_____

_____

_____

_____

Tracking Your Pursuit

Day 18

What was your mood today?

    a) Happy
    b) Sad
    c) Angry
    d) Other

Why did you feel this way?

What are you most thankful for today?

Tracking Your Pursuit

Did you achieve your goals for the day? Why or why not?

Daily Journal Entry

I STILL Want To Be A Mom

Tracking Your Pursuit

Day 19

What was your mood today?

    a) Happy
    b) Sad
    c) Angry
    d) Other

Why did you feel this way?

_____

_____

_____

_____

_____

_____

What are you most thankful for today?

_____

_____

_____

_____

_____

_____

I STILL Want To Be A Mom

Did you achieve your goals for the day? Why or why not?

Daily Journal Entry

Tracking Your Pursuit

Day 20

What was your mood today?

    a) Happy
    b) Sad
    c) Angry
    d) Other

Why did you feel this way?

_____

_____

_____

_____

_____

_____

What are you most thankful for today?

_____

_____

_____

_____

_____

_____

_____

Tracking Your Pursuit

Did you achieve your goals for the day? Why or why not?

Daily Journal Entry

I STILL Want To Be A Mom

Day 21

What was your mood today?

    a) Happy
    b) Sad
    c) Angry
    d) Other

Why did you feel this way?

_____
_____
_____
_____
_____
_____

What are you most thankful for today?

_____
_____
_____
_____
_____
_____

Did you achieve your goals for the day? Why or why not?

Daily Journal Entry

Tracking Your Pursuit

Day 22

What was your mood today?

    a) Happy
    b) Sad
    c) Angry
    d) Other

Why did you feel this way?

What are you most thankful for today?

Did you achieve your goals for the day? Why or why not?

Daily Journal Entry

I STILL Want To Be A Mom

Day 23

What was your mood today?

    a) Happy
    b) Sad
    c) Angry
    d) Other

Why did you feel this way?

What are you most thankful for today?

I STILL Want To Be A Mom

Did you achieve your goals for the day? Why or why not?

_____

_____

_____

_____

_____

Daily Journal Entry

_____

_____

_____

_____

_____

_____

_____

_____

_____

_____

_____

Tracking Your Pursuit

Day 24

What was your mood today?

    a) Happy
    b) Sad
    c) Angry
    d) Other

Why did you feel this way?

_____

_____

_____

_____

_____

_____

What are you most thankful for today?

_____

_____

_____

_____

_____

_____

Did you achieve your goals for the day? Why or why not?

Daily Journal Entry

I STILL Want To Be A Mom

Day 25

What was your mood today?

    a) Happy
    b) Sad
    c) Angry
    d) Other

Why did you feel this way?

What are you most thankful for today?

Did you achieve your goals for the day? Why or why not?

_____

_____

_____

_____

_____

_____

Daily Journal Entry

_____

_____

_____

_____

_____

_____

_____

_____

_____

_____

_____

_____

Tracking Your Pursuit

Day 26

What was your mood today?

    a) Happy
    b) Sad
    c) Angry
    d) Other

Why did you feel this way?

_____

_____

_____

_____

_____

_____

What are you most thankful for today?

_____

_____

_____

_____

_____

_____

Tracking Your Pursuit

Did you achieve your goals for the day? Why or why not?

Daily Journal Entry

I STILL Want To Be A Mom

Day 27

What was your mood today?

    a) Happy
    b) Sad
    c) Angry
    d) Other

Why did you feel this way?

What are you most thankful for today?

Did you achieve your goals for the day? Why or why not?

Daily Journal Entry

Tracking Your Pursuit

Day 28

What was your mood today?

    a) Happy
    b) Sad
    c) Angry
    d) Other

Why did you feel this way?

___

What are you most thankful for today?

___

Did you achieve your goals for the day? Why or why not?

Daily Journal Entry

I STILL Want To Be A Mom

Day 29

What was your mood today?

- a) Happy
- b) Sad
- c) Angry
- d) Other

Why did you feel this way?

_____

_____

_____

_____

_____

_____

What are you most thankful for today?

_____

_____

_____

_____

_____

_____

Did you achieve your goals for the day? Why or why not?

Daily Journal Entry

Tracking Your Pursuit

Day 30

What was your mood today?

- a) Happy
- b) Sad
- c) Angry
- d) Other

Why did you feel this way?

_____
_____
_____
_____
_____
_____

What are you most thankful for today?

_____
_____
_____
_____
_____
_____
_____

Did you achieve your goals for the day? Why or why not?

Daily Journal Entry

I STILL Want To Be A Mom

Chapter 10

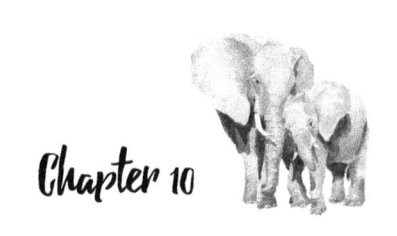

HELLO MOM

This chapter is meant to be read after you get pregnant.

Hello Mom,

Congratulations! You are officially pregnant. Hallelujah! I'm sure by now you've seen positive pregnancy tests, positive HCG results, and maybe even heard your little one's heartbeat. You have worked very hard and the moment you have been waiting for is finally here. You went from saying, "I will be a mom" to now saying, "OMG, I am really about to be a mom." In this entire book, I have referred to overcoming infertility as a journey, but in all actuality the journey has just begun. There is a new life growing inside of you and while you are excited, now you probably have new worries. Your mind is probably being filled with hundreds of "what ifs." Considering all you had to go through to get to this point, you may not feel all of the warm fuzziness in your heart that you see in the movies when a woman is pregnant. You may not feel a special bond with your baby right away and I am here to tell you that it is perfectly normal if you don't. Even if you don't feel anything, remember to use the tips you learned from the earlier chapters, mainly the ones about preparing your mind and perspective to help you stay positive. Since in knowing, from experience, that you will still have moments of fear and worry to overcome, I have included a pregnancy mantra to the end of this chapter that you can say daily to keep yourself focused on the positive throughout your pregnancy. Read it out loud in the mirror daily when you start out your day and when you end your day. That way when you wake up, you can shape your thoughts for the day and before you go to bed, you can have something positive on your mind. I want you to remember that just because you had a hard time getting or staying pregnant in the past, it doesn't mean something negative will happen this pregnancy. You will have a happy and healthy nine months. If you speak it enough, you will believe it.

> I want you to remember that just because you had a hard time getting or staying pregnant in the past, it doesn't mean something negative will happen this pregnancy.

Here are some other activities you can do to keep yourself occupied and encouraged during your pregnancy:

- If you have forged a relationship with ladies from an infertility support group, check back in periodically with ladies who are still trying to get pregnant and share inspirational thoughts with them from your story and answer questions they may have about the journey. This will help keep you smiling.
- If you haven't already done so, join a pregnancy-after-infertility support group or forum to have support from other ladies going through a similar experience.
- Try not to take insensitive comments to heart. Many people don't know what to say when they find out you

got pregnant using infertility treatments. Sometimes people are not trying to be rude; they just don't know what to say.
- If you find that you are battling depression and unable to manage your emotions, talk to your doctor. It has been a rough journey and just because you are pregnant doesn't mean that all of your negative feelings and thoughts will just go away.
- Take a vacation or weekend getaway at some point during your pregnancy. The second trimester may be best.
- Write down questions for your OB-GYN prior to the appointments so you don't forget what you were going to say. There are no silly questions. This is your pregnancy and your baby, so if you have concerns, don't be ashamed to bring them up.
- If you are uneasy and worried about miscarriage constantly, you may want to invest in a home doppler. You can find an inexpensive one online. Be advised that you may not be able to find the heartbeat easily using one until the second trimester, so if you think struggling to find it will cause you more stress, don't get one.

—Pregnancy Mantra—

I am so excited to be pregnant. I am thrilled that I will have the opportunity to be a mom. I have been waiting for this moment for a long time.

I am going to be happy throughout my pregnancy.

I am going to be thankful throughout my pregnancy.

I am going to be a good mom.

I am going to take care of my body, eat right, and get proper rest.

I am beautiful.

I am fearfully and wonderfully made.

I am going to enjoy every moment of this pregnancy.

I am so glad that I did not give up during my journey, even though I experienced many failures and heartaches along the way.

I have fought so hard to get to this place, and I will not let anything discourage me.

I will not complain.

I will not focus on past failures.

I will not speak negatively because I realize that my words shape my mood.

I will not worry because I realize that my worries are usually about situations that are beyond my control.

I will not be afraid because I realize that my fears are usually about situations occurring that haven't even happened or won't happen.

I know that fears are fake exaggerations affecting my reality, and I will not allow myself to concentrate on them.

I will practice replacing negative thoughts with positive ones until it gets easier and easier to think positively.

I will not be down.

I will not be depressed.

I will not blame myself.

I will not blame others.

I will choose joy instead of pain.

I will choose love instead of fear.

I will choose expectation instead of worry.

I will do what I can and not worry about what I can't.

I will surround myself with people who encourage me and promote positivity in my life.

When no one else is around to encourage me, I will encourage myself. After all, I have been able to make it this far.

Nothing can stop me. I am a conqueror.

I am strong. I can do this.

I will survive this journey.

I will have a healthy pregnancy.

I will deliver a healthy baby.

I will have a happy, healthy, and safe delivery.

I will get to take my baby home with me this time.

I can't wait to hold my baby in my arms for the first time.

This thought makes me smile because as I say this, I am literally visualizing my baby in my arms. Wow, MY baby in MY arms.

My heart is smiling. My face is smiling. The love I feel for this growing life inside of me overpowers any negative thoughts.

I am filled with excitement, because I am so much closer to this moment today than I was yesterday.

I am so excited to be pregnant. I am thrilled that I will have the opportunity to be a mom. I have been waiting for this moment for a long time and it is finally happening. Yes, it is finally happening.

I am a mom.

REFERENCES

1. Amanapu, G. (2016, September 12). *The Pregnant Dog And Elephant: Motivational Story*. Retrieved from Linkedin: https://www.linkedin.com/pulse/pregnant-dog-elephant-motivational-story-girish-amanapu

2. Office On Women's Health . (2018, March 30). *Infertility* . Retrieved from U.S. Department of Health & Human Services : https://www.womenshealth.gov/a-z-topics/infertility

3. Resolve . (2018, March 30). *Secondary Infertility* . Retrieved from Resolve : https://resolve.org/infertility-101/medical-conditions/secondary-infertility/

4. Resolve. (2018, March 30). *Fast Facts*. Retrieved from Resolve: https://resolve.org/infertility-101/what-is-infertility/fast-facts/

5. Christodoulou, E. (2013, March 9). *Career Guide*. Retrieved from MyStarJob: http://mystarjob.com/articles/story.aspx?file=/2013/3/9/mystarjob_careerguide/12763006&sec=mystarjob_careerguide

6. James, W. (2018, March 30). Retrieved from BrainyQuote: https://www.brainyquote.com/quotes/william_james_385478

Lightning Source UK Ltd.
Milton Keynes UK
UKHW010411230520
363730UK00003B/822